THE A-Z OF
APPLIED
QUALITY
FOR CLINICAL MANAGERS IN HOSPITALS

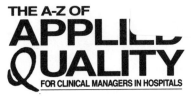

To

Melanie Brooks.

with best wishes from

Nan Kemp

September 1994

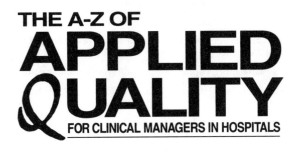

THE A-Z OF
APPLIED
QUALITY
FOR CLINICAL MANAGERS IN HOSPITALS

Denise Barnett

Professional Adviser in the Health Section of the
National Audit Office

and

Nan Kemp

Quality Assurance Adviser in Health Care

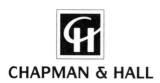

CHAPMAN & HALL

London · Glasgow · Weinheim · New York · Tokyo · Melbourne · Madras

Published by Chapman & Hall, 2–6 Boundary Row, London SE1 8HN, UK

Chapman & Hall, 2–6 Boundary Row, London SE1 8HN, UK

Blackie Academic & Professional, Wester Cleddens Road, Bishopbriggs, Glasgow G64 2NZ, UK

Chapman & Hall GmbH, Pappelallee 3, 69469 Weinheim, Germany

Chapman & Hall USA., One Penn Plaza, 41st Floor, New York NY 10119, USA

Chapman & Hall Japan, ITP-Japan, Kyowa Building, 3F, 2-2-1 Hirakawacho, Chiyoda-ku, Tokyo 102, Japan

Chapman & Hall Australia, Thomas Nelson Australia, 102 Dodds Street, South Melbourne, Victoria 3205, Australia

Chapman & Hall India, R. Seshadri, 32 Second Main Road, CIT East, Madras 600 035, India

Distributed in the USA and Canada by Singular Publishing Group Inc., 4284 41st Street, San Diego, California 92105

First Edition 1994

© 1994 Denise Barnett and Nan Kemp

Typeset in 10/12 Palatino by Florencetype

Printed in Great Britain by St Edmundsbury Press, Bury St Edmunds, Suffolk

ISBN 0 412 56930 2   1 56593 376 1 (USA)

A catalogue record for this book is available from the British Library

Library of Congress Catalog Card Number: 94-71820

∞ Printed on permanent acid-free text paper, manufactured in accordance with ANSI/NISO Z39.48-1992 and ANSI/NISO Z39.48-1984 (Permanence of Paper).

Contents

W

X/Y

Z

Preface

The clinical manager in hospital manages the day-to-day activities within a clinical area which may be a clinical directorate. The professional background of the manager varies; doctors, nurses, midwives, physiotherapists, radiographers, administrators and others may take the lead.

The main focus of the clinical manager in hospital is normally ward activity. This A—Z reference book acknowledges this but also covers activities that may be devolved to the directorate. As nurses still form the bulk of the workforce within the wards, some of the topics provide information for the manager with a limited knowledge of nursing.

Clinical managers are busy people, with many competing calls on their time. The authors hope that the 'skip and dip' format will help the reader to speedily select topics for information or ideas for improving quality. References and suggestions of further reading provide opportunities to pursue an interest to greater depth. Where possible, the shorter texts and articles have been chosen.

There is no single recipe for success in achieving a health service of high quality. Each manager has to assess the starting point of the present team, to assemble a vision of what could be achieved and to plan the route to making it a reality. The responsibility may at times seem overwhelming. Acting on one topic a month should be manageable and enhance the quality over a year.

Whilst Ms Barnett is employed by the National Audit Office, the views expressed in this book are her own and not those of the National Audit Office.

Acknowledgements

This book is based on our practical experience and the action learning entailed in experimenting with different approaches. Thanks are due to everyone who has helped us over the years.

In preparing this book we gratefully acknowledge the willing help of colleagues who read and critiqued the early drafts: Rosie and Peter Cunliffe, Terri Fox, Sarah Kemp, Roger Le Voir, Becky Malby and Tony Pepper. Their different perspectives were very helpful.

There were others who patiently answered our questions and provided advice. In particular we thank Jo Beschi, Sue Brown, Mary Godfree, Gillian Heslop, Jane Martin, Barbara Milburn, Chris Nyam and Eileen Richardson.

Thanks are also due to Gillian and Nick Heslop who were generous enough to let us work in the comfort and quiet of their home on several occasions.

Finally, we would like to thank Tom Keighly for his help in the preparation of the manuscript.

Introduction

Hospital staff are now under pressure not only to deliver a high-quality service but also to demonstrate that they do so consistently.

This is particularly tough when education and training in quality management is not readily available. Those working in the new clinical directorate structures, from whatever professional background, also face the problem of overall responsibility for quality of care and treatment provided by staff from a range of clinical disciplines.

The management of health care provided by the NHS is undergoing a period of rapid change. New management structures, roles and relationships are being created with each change of chief executive. A decade of emphasis on efficiency with throughput has been followed by an increased emphasis on quality. The setting of standards and assessment of later achievement have become important for all the public services as resources shrink and demands increase. Value for money is examined by the Audit Commission and the National Audit Office and managers are expected to examine whether their findings apply locally.

Television, newspapers and magazines have helped to educate and raise the expectations of the public about the quality of care and treatment that could be provided. Patients expect choice, consultation and explanation. The professional organizations seek high-quality education and training environments for their members.

Total quality management, where the whole organization is involved, along with its customers (i.e. HAs and GPs) and consumers (i.e. patients, their relatives and carers) is being promoted. Staff and patients are slowly being empowered to shape the service, so it becomes more effective, user-friendly, budget-conscious and uses information technology, all to demonstrate increased value for the public money it spends. Clinical managers have to take the lead, with support from those with more technical expertise in audit and quality assurance.

Further reading

Ham, C. (1985) From efficiency monitoring to quality assurance: the development of monitoring in the NHS. *Hospital and Health Service Review* , **81,** 3, 110–113.

Teeling Smith, G. (1989) *Measurement and Management in the NHS,* Report No. 91, Office of Health Economics, London.

A

ACCIDENTS

Quality and safety should be synonymous. All managers have a responsibility for the prevention of accidents in their area. Every employee has a responsibility to behave in a manner that keeps people and the environment safe. A high-quality service also concerns itself with the 'near miss' – trying to build preventative action into daily activities.

Every manager has a responsibility to ensure that their staff know about and have access to the policies and procedures that relate to safety. It is helpful to have an accident prevention checklist to guide new staff members and those staff who visit clinical areas on a regular basis.

The Health and Safety at Work Act [1] sets out the responsibilities of employers to ensure that premises, equipment and systems of work are safe and without risk to health. There are also supporting acts and regulations that deal with particular hazards and types of work. With the implementation of the Regulations for Control of Substances Hazardous to Health (COSHH) [2], inspections are required of all substances kept within the premises. This is to ensure that no hazardous substances are stored unnecessarily and to check if they are still needed and stored safely. If staff are using substances that are particularly dangerous, they will need to undergo regular medical health checks. Staff must be provided with, and they must use, the appropriate protective clothing and the correct equipment.

When an accident occurs, the person in charge at the time must take prompt action to prevent any further damage or danger occurring. She or he must record the facts as they appear and look for the cause. A record of the details about the accident, the action taken and the outcome should be entered in an accident register.

When injury has occurred the person in charge must not allow his or her natural sympathy for the injured person to overshadow the need for a careful analysis of the facts. Any individual(s) involved should, if they are able, write out a statement. They may be shocked and unable to give a coherent account. Some people may wish to forget the facts. It is however important to establish as soon as possible, exactly what caused the accident. Reports should be written as soon after the event as possible. People have been known to change their perception of the event and even blame others or change their story after an accident. Counselling should be available to any member of staff, patient or visitor who has been involved in an accident.

The Safety Representative should be contacted as soon as possible following the initial analysis. It may be necessary to take photographs or to make sketches and impound equipment. There will be a need to review the events leading up to the accident and the action taken. No one should make 'off-the-cuff' statements or jump to premature conclusions since such actions can do harm to individuals and misguide any enquiry.

In the event of a severe accident, the Health and Safety Executive will want to know when checks were carried out and what action was taken to remedy faults and will wish to see the relevant reports.

Every manager should be concerned about all accidents. It is wise to check the accident reports routinely and take note of trends. An early warning of potential problems may need to be taken to a quality team meeting.

It is also helpful to hold a regular seminar to review trends, clustering of accidents, incidents and near misses. This gives an opportunity to pool ideas on improvements. The group activity can increase staff commitment to accurate, detailed recording. Analysis of the hospital forms and any additional material collected for local interest can form the basis of the discussion. Having identified the probable cause, an action plan should be drawn up. Quality circles can be helpful if there are a series of near misses or accidents.

An annual health and safety audit for all aspects of safety maintenance and accident prevention should be carried out and include:

- safety training requirements;
- structure of the building and defects noted, e.g. bulging ceilings;
- temperature, light and ventilation;
- access and egress to all areas;

- condition of equipment and when it is checked and was last checked;
- fire prevention;
- infection-control procedures, including universal precautions;
- housekeeping, including the correct disposal of waste clinical material and used equipment.

These reports must be signed by the ward manager and the safety representative.

The annual audit is also a good time to check whether the area has hazards to staff from drunk, drugged or confused patients or visitors e.g. heavy ashtrays or items that can be picked up and thrown. Where staff see patients alone or if they may work alone after hours, it is also important to provide a system that enables them to summon help.

References
1. Health and Safety Commission *Health and Safety at Work Act, 1974*, HMSO, London.
2. Statutory Instrument No. 1657. The Control of Substances Hazardous to Health Regulations. 1988, HMSO, London.

Further reading
Editorial (1990) Report that accident. *Nursing Times*, **86**, 13, 53–54.
Gibbs, J. (1990) Action on the environment; disposal of waste. *Nursing Times*, **86**, 51, 34–35.
Health and Safety Commission, Health Services Advisory Committee (1982) *The Safe Disposal of Clinical Waste in 1981*, HMSO, London.
Health and Safety Executive (1986) *A Guide to Reporting of Injuries, Diseases and Dangerous Occurrences Regulations (RIDDOR)*, 1985, Health and safety series booklet HS(R) 23, HMSO, London.
Simpson, D. and Simpson, G.W. (1991) *The COSHH Regulations: A Practical Guide*, The Royal Society of Chemistry, Cambridge, London.

Information source
The Health and Safety Executive (HSE, telephone 071-243-6385), produce a wide range of leaflets.

ADVERTISING FOR STAFF

A wise manager acknowledges that the current staff are the directorate's best advertisement. It can be useful to get staff to list honestly the good points about working in the wards and the difficulties, without mentioning names. The results can then be analysed and a plan developed to deal with the problems.

An advertisement for staff can also act as a marketing opportunity for the hospital, directorate and ward. It therefore needs careful thought and usually some professional help. An effective advertisement produces enquiries only from those who are appropriately qualified. A massive response usually indicates a poorly focused advert. Respondents should have already performed through self-selection the first sifting out of unsuitable candidates.

It may be possible at one interview session to find more good candidates than there are currently vacant posts. Start a waiting list of those eager to join the team when the next suitable vacancy occurs.

The following items form a useful briefing pack for the advertising agency:

- the list of strengths and difficulties identified by the staff;
- the action plan;
- the mission statement of the unit, directorate and ward;
- a list of the special qualities required in the candidates at all levels for posts that may fall vacant during the coming year;
- essential professional qualifications.

Dates should be arranged for informal visits when team members will be available to show the candidates around the hospital. Include the first name of the person to be contacted about the posts. Jane Smith sounds more friendly than Mrs J. Smith.

Find out what kinds of advert the present agency can produce if given a free hand. Central control by the Personnel Department who try to do most of the design before contacting the agency can lead to poor marketing of the hospital.

If the present agency has grown complacent ask others to tender for your work and submit examples. Be prepared to invest 80% of the directorate's advertising budget on one good piece of copy and graphics. The person who will deal with the advert could be invited to visit the hospital and meet the present staff. Send the briefing pack to the selected agency with details of the vacant posts. Leave them to design the advert. Respect their expertise. Promise the agency that it will be 'run as written', only correcting factual errors.

Run the advert in the national or local press according to the need to bring in advanced skills or to find local staff who can work the shift times required.

Arrange a meeting with the advertising agency who drew up the advert to discuss the response. Provide a breakdown of the age range, skills offered, home locality, reason for the interest for all those who wrote for details. Work out together how the next advert can be made even more effective.

If the response was good, the manager can share the information with the personnel department. If the wards have a steady turnover of staff, the manager should consider sharing a block advert with other directorates, once a month, using a consistent style, in one or two newspapers or journals. If the directorate has a high turnover this is usually a sign of work problems. Potential respondents know this and will not apply for posts.

Further reading

Edis, M. and Smith, A. (1988) Advertising by design. *Nursing Times*, **85**, 30, 41–43.

Hackett, P., Schofield, P. and Armstrong, M. (1982) *The Daily Telegraph Recruitment Handbook*, 2nd edn., Kogan Page, London.

ADVOCACY

Advocacy is defined as: 'pleading support of' [1]. It is part of caring and is not separate from ongoing care. It is needed when the patient is unable, for whatever reason, to speak up for him or herself.

> Advocacy is concerned with promoting and safeguarding the well-being and interest of patients and clients. It is not concerned with conflict for its own sake.
>
> UKCC, 1989

Advocacy is ethically based and given the various value systems, expectations and coping mechanisms of patients and those significant to them; it is not something to be undertaken lightly. The values of patients and the health carers may be in conflict or just different from each other; this can present problems.

It is important for a quality service to look at how, and if, effective patient advocacy is being practised by health care staff. One may feel that protection of the patients' rights is implicit in the

philosophy of health carers without having to implement a
specific system of advocacy. However, there are reported
incidents of poor practice and poor communication, with little
or no informed consent for the patient or those significant to him
or her.

Any manager wishing to develop a specific system of advocacy
should consider the implications and the responsibility it carries.
An initial enquiry could include reading around the subject and
a visit to an area where advocacy is being carried out effectively.
Discussion between members of the team should take place to get
their views and suggestions. As with any system, it should be
well-planned, understood by all those likely to be involved and
monitored carefully.

Consideration of the following points may be helpful:

- Does the philosophy of the directorate acknowledge and
  reinforce the rights of patients in daily practice?
- Potential advocates and the manager must care about people,
  believe in and understand the principal underpinning advocacy and the inherent difficulties.
- Will the directorate be able to cope with these problems that
  seem to have no easy solutions, e.g. the patient's right to
  refuse life-saving measures?
- An advocate should know themselves, have confidence
  without conceit or arrogance.
- Advocates should be articulate.
- At times the advocate may have to be brave and risk
  offending colleagues.
- Will the advocates be able to understand the patients'
  problems, their background, needs and, where possible, their
  expectations?
- Who is to teach/facilitate the would-be advocates?
- Is there a counselling system available to staff?

The advocate must also be sensitive to the needs of those people
close to the patient. The principles of informed consent have to
be understood. 'Taking the right of decision away from the
patients or relatives should only occur in the rarest of cases' [2].
The advocate should also appreciate the rights of colleagues but
not put them before those of the patient. One of the reasons for
avoiding advocacy is that too often staff are afraid to speak up
for fear of offending a colleague.

There are dangers. That is why the principles of advocacy must be understood by all the team members to ensure that the actions of the advocate are neither misinterpreted nor misguided.

Patient advocacy may involve risk-taking and, at times, could be at odds with the rules of the directorate. It may cause conflict between professionals and professions. Those who become advocates, separate from their everyday work, should also be able to give up the role if they cannot cope with it. Some health professionals may see a specific system of advocacy as an erosion of their relationship with the patients, their status, responsibility and professionalism.

The purpose of advocacy should not be forgotten. It must not become yet another means of controlling people.

There are some long-stay areas where staff have been using a specific system of advocacy for several years. In some areas such as those helping people with learning disabilities, self-advocacy groups have been set up [3, 4].

Citizen advocacy has existed in Britain since 1981 with the advent of 'Advocacy Alliance' in London. Since then many projects have sprung up around the country [5]. Citizen advocacy occurs when a private citizen befriends a disadvantaged person and learns to represent their true interest [5]. It can occur both in the community and in institutions. There are positive gains with this system; there are also problems to be overcome before the system works effectively in all areas.

Effective patient allocation in hospital will facilitate informed consent or refusal as the patient and health professional can openly discuss issues. The patient may be able to nominate a relative or friend to act as his or her representative or, where necessary, have the professional act as an informed friend. Informed consent is one of the criteria for high-quality care.

Quality in practice

Mr Smith had been in the hospital ward for several days; his family knew he might require emergency cardiac surgery. His wife was sitting with him. One daughter was studying in the hospital library, the other was 200 miles away. Suddenly his condition worsened. The medical decision was to operate. The room became busy as the final tests were completed and Mr Smith prepared for theatre.

His wife was frightened; she tried to be inconspicuous and appear calm. She covered up her feelings in case they distracted the staff in caring for her husband.

Then Rose, his primary nurse, came into the room. She asked Mrs Smith how she was bearing up – Mrs Smith said 'fine'. Rose quietly and calmly told her what the procedure would entail, explaining she could stay with her husband for most of the time before he was transferred to the operating theatre. Rose had already contacted Susan in the hospital library and she was on her way over. Rose explained that the other daughter was being contacted by the ward clerk so that Mrs Smith could talk with her.

Rose also suggested that Mrs Smith might wish to speak to the surgeon – he was on his way from the theatre – Mrs Smith felt she should not bother him but when he arrived Rose introduced him and prompted Mrs Smith to ask questions. Rose also introduced the anaesthetist. Mrs Smith found both men kind and answered her questions, prompted by Rose. The nurse suggested that Mrs Smith and her daughter should walk part of the way to the theatre alongside Mr Smith.

This caring nurse looked after both the patient and his family. She recognized that the family were close and that they were determined not to be a nuisance to the staff. In the crisis she temporarily took over the decision-making for them, acting as an advocate in ensuring that the whole family's unspoken needs were met.

References

1. Sykes, J.B. (ed.)(1988) *The Concise Oxford Dictionary*, 7th edn., Oxford University Press, Oxford.
2. UKCC (1989) *Exercising Accountability*, A UKCC Advisory Document, UKCC, London.
3. Lindsay, A. and Marler, R. (1989) Unrealistic expectations? *Nursing Times*, **85**, 42, 33–34.
4. Butler, K. (1987) Citizen advocacy in action. *New Society*, **80**, April 24, 2.
5. Branch, R. (1985) Citizen advocacy. *Nursing Mirror*, **160**, 14, 31–32.

Further reading

Cornwall, J. and Gordon, P. (1984) *Experiment in Advocacy. The Hackney Multi-Ethnic Women's Health Project,* Kings Fund, London.

Department of Health (1980) *Inequalities in Health,* HMSO, London.

Department of Health (1991) *The Patient's Charter,* HMSO, London.

Kohnke, M.F. (1980) *Advocacy, Risk and Reality,* Mosby, New York.

McSweeney, P. (1990) Accountability in nursing practice. *Nursing Standard,* **4**, 18, 30–31.

Oswald, R. (1990) The Health Service Ombudsman. *Journal of the Royal Association for Disability and Rehabilitation,* **Spring edn.,** 37.

Salvage, J. (1985) *The Politics in Nursing,* Macmillan, London.

UKCC (1993) *Code of Professional Conduct for the Nurse, Midwife and Health Visitor* UK Central Council for Nursing, Midwifery and Health Visiting, London.

Winkler, F. (1987) Consumerism in health care: beyond the supermarket model. *Policy and Politics,* **15**, 1, 1–8.

ALLOCATION OF STAFF

The aim is for continuity of contact between the same staff and patients. Allocation to a geographical area of a ward, with a group of patients at a mixed dependency level for variety, is helpful for student nurses. Such allocations can last for 4 weeks or more provided that there are registered nurses to supervise and teach.

Qualified nurses allocated to a high-dependency group that has a rapid throughput of patients may require a change in allocation to a less stressful area after 2–3 weeks. Internal rotation to different patient groups in a ward, between wards and to night duty can be stimulating. This can be of particular importance in a long-stay ward. Staff in other disciplines, such as therapists and junior doctors, may also find particular patient groups stressful. Thought should be given to suitable means to relieve their problems.

Team and primary nursing offer continuity. The ward sister then acts as co-ordinator and consultant in nursing to the ward staff.

Primary nursing is now well documented. Briefly it is when a qualified nurse acts as the primary nurse, responsible for co-ordinating and prescribing nursing care throughout the patient's stay in the ward. The named nurse is now a feature of the 'Patient's Charter'. The other qualified nurses or senior student nurses act as associate nurses and take responsibility for providing care in the absence of the primary nurse. Junior students and nursing auxiliaries/care assistants provide help in following the plan of care prescribed by the primary nurse.

This system requires a high ratio of qualified nurses; they also become eligible for the higher clinical grades. The level of responsibility is increased and the nurse and patient will benefit from additional clinical preparation and skills development.

Primary nursing requires that any computer-based staff-allocation system takes into account the patient groupings; if not uneven workloads may result. Topping-up the nurse hours with bank and agency staff as associate nurses does not affect the care plan continuity but it can be expensive.

Team nursing may be administratively easier to organize. A qualified nurse leads a team consisting of other qualified nurses, students and nursing auxiliaries. Each ward is divided into patient groups with its allocated nursing team. The ideal is to have one team subdivided to cover all three shifts, with internal rotation to the night shift. Inexperienced qualified nurses can receive support with the team leader acting as preceptor.

Staff rosters are a prime target for the computer. Too often the programmers see rosters as a simple task for a spreadsheet and ignore the skill mix and grade mix requirements, as well as the continuity of primary nursing. The organization of the ward also requires flexibility to cope with consultants' rounds, operating days, meetings, patient outings and admission days.

Software should be selected with these requirements in mind. The variations in workload during the day need to be reflected in a shift-by-shift analysis of the average hours of care required by patients on each day of the week. The aim should be to have at least 85% of these average patient care hours covered by a core of permanent staff on the day shifts and for 100% cover on night duty. A top-up system should be arranged for boosting the day shifts with flexible hours, part-time, bank or agency time booked for the next two shifts, according to the predictions based on the current workload. Such flexibility is more difficult to arrange for night shifts and this lies behind the recommended 100% core staffing. In small wards there may be a minimum number of staff required to maintain safety, irrespective of low patient-care hours requirements.

A good system will be able to imitate some of the balancing of patients' needs with available nursing skills that the experienced ward sister achieves when compiling a manual duty roster and allocating from the staff on duty at the start of a shift.

Altering traditional shift patterns, to improve the quality of patient care by improving the use of staff time, needs careful handling. Female staff often have to adjust child care and house-keeping with shift times. Travel and the risk of violence on dark nights may also require new arrangements. Special duty payments for unsociable hours may be affected. It is also important to ensure staff will be able to balance work periods with leisure and home-making.

Logging the information about the patients' requirements in terms of hours of nursing and other staff time, and allowing staff greater flexibility in deciding how to meet them, may give a higher quality than imposing change as some hospitals have tried to do. It also means different starting and finishing times among wards in the same directorate or hospital. The manage-ment accountant's help in costing such proposals should be sought. It may be helpful to cost several options.

The manager should monitor the resulting rosters for fairness in the allocation of weekends and evenings off-duty, taking charge and of busy times. The rosters for all disciplines need similar scrutiny as resentment and charges of discrimination can follow poor distribution. The senior person who always elects to work the weekends or extra time may create disquiet among the team. Income and pension boosting from such action may also be a sign of loss of commitment to the job and to quality.

Further reading

Audit Commission (1991) *The Virtue of Patients: Making the Best Use of Nursing Resources*, HMSO, London.

Bergen, A. (1992) Care management in community care; concepts, prac-tices and implications for nursing. *Journal of Advanced Nursing*, **17**, 9, 1106–13.

Black, F. (ed.) (1992) *Primary Nursing: An Introductory Guide*, Kings Fund Centre, London.

Cabell, C. (1992) The efficacy of primary nursing as a foundation for patient advocacy: nursing practice. *Nursing Standard*, **5**, 3.

Department of Health (1993) *A Vision for the Future. The Nursing Midwifery and Health Visiting Contribution to Health and Health Care*, NHS Management Executive, Leeds.

Eaves, D. (1992) Case mix management. *Senior Nurse*, **12**, 3, 8–10.

Hancock C. (1992) The named nurse concept. *Nursing Standard*, **16**, 17, 16–18.

Lear, G., Morris, G., Parnel, M. and Wharne, S. (1991) Care management: responding to the need. *Nursing Times*, **87**, 50, 24–26.

Procter, S. (1991) Patient allocation and the unqualified learner nurse. Occasional paper. *Nursing Times*, **87**, 43, 46–48.

Royal College of Nursing (1992) *Issues in Nursing and Health: Approaches to Nursing Care, Paper 13*, RCN, London.

AUDIT

Audit was originally a financial term referring to the official examination of accounts. In the field of quality it was used initially for the examination of written or computer-based records, to examine the workflow, numbers treated and so on.

It may also be used in the NHS to mean the examination of clinical records to find indicators of the quality of service offered. Thus the meaning has become less precise and the term may be used to describe one or more of the following activities: the checking of standards; criteria; objectives; or outcomes in order to obtain an index of the quality of service. Occasionally it is used to mean the gathering of information by asking questions, checking records and observing clinical practice, the environment or the use of resources.

AUDIT OF CLINICAL AREAS

The term 'audit' may be applied to the work of one discipline such as 'medical audit' or 'nursing audit'. Clinical audit is a co-operative, multi-professional assessment of the efficacy, social acceptability and economic efficiency of the care and treatment of patients with a specified disease, disorder or disability. It may focus on the process or outcome of individual components or on the total care experience.

Clinical audit involves all the professionals pooling their evaluations of the care and treatment of individual patients, or examining selected aspects for a group of patients.

Audit is the examination of records with an evaluation of the findings and a plan of action on the issues raised when debating them. It starts with the basic assumption that if an action is not recorded, it was not carried out. Simple workload statistics can give information about lengths of stay. The frequency of complications about admissions or infections can be counted and compared with the total patients cared for over an agreed period.

Critical incident reviews can be very useful – it is not just the airline pilots who can learn from the 'near miss'. The quality of the service and care can be improved by spotting when an early intervention would stop the situation deteriorating into a serious problem.

Established multi-disciplinary teams may be able to move into clinical audit without first going through the uni-disciplinary audit stage. Clinical audit requires trust and a focus on improving patient care, not point-scoring between professional groups.

The audit group should meet regularly every 4–6 weeks. At first, new groups may go through several stages, identified by Benedikter [1]:

- **procedure writers** – watch for wording in the present tense, lots of detail and 'needs to be observed' phrases;
- **patient's ombudsman** – the group uses day-to-day experience and considers plenty of 'what ifs. . .';
- **process criteria writers** – the group focuses on detail, not on the key topics;
- **uni-disciplinary criteria writers**.

Audit groups fail if they:

- act only as medical record-completion committees;
- use personal opinion, not facts.

Once the group is well established, rotate part of the membership each year so that new perspectives are introduced and more staff benefit from the experience of scrutinizing clinical work.

Devising an agreed protocol for the treatment and care of patients with specific diseases can act as a focus for discussion and provide a template for audit clerks to review a sample of the clinical notes to identify if all the important steps have been carried out.

When selecting diseases for such protocols, it may be helpful to chose from those diseases that cause patients the most discomfort. The clear guidelines of the protocol help reduce the stress on junior staff, struggling to bring relief to the patient. The work on sickle cell crises by City and Hackney DHA is one example. The increased pain control, patient involvement and audit feedback led to improvement in patient care and greater confidence among junior doctors and nurses.

Once the professionals have identified and agreed the criteria to be considered, the task can be delegated to trained clerks from the medical records department or those employed by the audit and quality assurance team. Their reports to the clinical team on the rate of omissions in the sample records will provide the starting point for professional involvement and action plans.

Clinical audit needs additional time for data collection, for its analysis and to help initiate the agreed changes. It may be necessary to adjust the workloads of those involved in the audit group meetings as well as employing staff to support the new activity.

The audit officers, who do the 'legwork' of data collection, and the information department staff who may provide assistance with the analysis and presentation should be acknowledged. Their interest and enthusiasm for future work can be enhanced by providing a summary of the action taken by the audit group. Presentation of the data at audit meetings is important. Numbers need to be presented in a visual form for easy absorption. There are now spreadsheet packages, which run on a small personal computer, that can turn data into graphs, pie charts or histograms at the touch of a few buttons.

On finding problems, the focus should be on agreeing remedial action [1]. The audit group should be asked:

- Who should be doing what?
- Why aren't they doing it? Is it because of:
    the tools?
    the forms?
    the policy or procedures?
    differences in beliefs or priorities?
    insufficient time or skilled staff?
    inadequate communication, especially between shifts?
    physical limitations in the building or the ward?
- What is in it for the staff if they don't get it right?
- Could they do it if their lives depended on it?
- What existing practices are there to prevent the problem from occurring?
- Why are the currently recommended practices ineffective or not followed?

Where a deviation from acceptable practice is found it should be referred to the relevant discipline so the process can be investigated and new standards set.

A record should be kept of who attended, the topics discussed and the decisions reached. The identity of patients and staff involved in their care should not be given. Confidentiality of patient details is essential.

There will always be a place for uni-disciplinary audit as an educational tool. Diagnostic departments need to carry out quality control; pathology and radiology departments can also make a significant contribution to the audit of care and clinical treatment of patients. They should be invited to join the audit group.

The Royal Colleges have compiled guidelines for medical audit and standard setting, which provide useful ideas for getting started. Computer-based clinical records aid rapid extraction of specific items for audit and some American systems are being adapted for use in the UK. The Department of Health has made money available to the NHS for medical and nursing audit systems that can also be used for clinical audit.

Reference

1. Benedikter, H. (1977) *From Nursing Audit to Multidisciplinary Audit*, National League for Nursing, New York.

Further reading

Black, N., Chappel, J., Dalziel, M. and Spilby, J. (1989) Step by step to audit. *Health Service Journal*, **February 2**, 40–41.

Department of Health (1989). *Medical Audit: Guidance for Hospital Clinicians on the Use of Computers*, HMSO, London.

NHS Management Executive (1994) *Clinical Audit 1994/5 and beyond*, EL (94) 20, Department of Health, Leeds.

Jones S.M. (1990) Clinical audit in general surgery. *International Journal of Health Care Quality Assurance*, **3**, 6, 17–20.

Salvage, J. (1990) Promoting good practice. *Nursing Standard*, **4**, 41, 52–53.

Stevens, G., and Bennett, J. (1989) Clinical audit – occurrence screening for quality assurance. *Health Services Management*, **85**, 4, 178–81.

Other resources

Teaching materials are available from the NHS Executive entitled 'Framework for Audit of Nursing Services' and 'Nursing Care Audit Teaching Notes'.

The *British Medical Journal* has contained regular articles entitled 'Audit in Practice' and 'Audit in Person'.

AUDIT OF NURSING EDUCATION AREAS

Colleges of Nursing and Midwifery are required to audit student learning areas annually, or more frequently if a ward is not reaching the required standard:

> At the highest level the Principal has authority delegated by the National Boards, which allows for units to be removed from the lists of suitable learning environments. [1]

The audit protocol is usually developed by teachers and clinical nurses, working together. They are guided by the requirements of the National Board [2] and the learning facilities in the clinical area.

Some standards and criteria are laid down by the national boards. For example, the standard statement with respect to practical placement (of students) from the English National Board is 'The quality of care and facilities provided for clients/patients must be such as to provide optimum learning to take place.' One of the criteria reads 'A minimum of one appropriately qualified first-level nurse must be available in a ward or department, to supervise students on each shift.'

The student nurse education audit covers a wide range of subjects, ranging from the philosophy of care, the learning climate, staffing levels, the method of organizing care, to whether the mentor system is working effectively. It would also have a criterion that referred to the ward learning objectives that had been set by the ward nursing staff.

It is necessary that all managers and ward sisters in the learning area are aware of the content of the audit document. They need to be sure that they are able to meet the requirements. If they are in doubt, a meeting should be arranged with a member of the college staff to discuss what is involved.

The audit is carried out by a nurse teacher and a member of the clinical staff. Results are processed and given, with recommendations, to the ward sister, who carries the responsibility for these results. The subsequent audit checks that the recommendations have been implemented. If an area receives an unsatisfactory report, the audit may be repeated in 3 or 6 months. The manager and ward sister should be positive, analysing the findings, identifying the good and looking for reasons for the unsatisfactory findings. For example: has the patient group changed? Has the work pattern altered? Have the staff sufficient resources to carry out effective teaching? Do staff have the right information and staffing to enable them to implement an effective patient allocation system? Are staff given the chance to attend appropriate courses and are such courses available? Are the ward learning objectives valid and readily accessible to students?

The manager and ward sister should ask themselves the following questions:

- Why did the situation arise in the first place?
- How can it be corrected?
- How can it be prevented from occurring again?

The ward sister should develop the action plan to overcome the identified weaknesses. If the solution lies outside the sister's and manager's control, the problem should be discussed with the appropriate teacher from the college, the director of the unit and if required, a more senior manager.

References

1. Kershaw, B. (1990) Clinical credibility and nurse teachers: Supplement 'A Strategy for Nursing'. *Nursing Standard*, 4, 51, 46–47.
2. English National Board (1989) *Regulations and guidelines for the approval of institutions and courses*, English National Board, London.

Further reading

Burnard, P. (1990) Is anyone here a mentor? *Nursing Standard*, 4, 37, 46.

Kemp, N. and Richardson, E. (1990) *Quality Assurance in Nursing Practice*, ch. 7, Butterworth-Heinemann, Oxford.

Nicklen, P. and Kenworthy, N. (1987) Educational audit. *Senior Nurse*, 7, 1, 22–24.

Orr, R. (1990) Developing an audit system. *Senior Nurse*, 10, 9, 14–15.

Shailer, B. (1990) Clinical learning environment audit (student nurses). *Nurse Education Today*, 10, 3, 220–27.

Spouse, J. (1990) Nurse-education issues: performance indicators. *Nursing Times*, 86, 6, 73–74.

B

BUDGETS

Many budgets are drawn up on no more that what was spent in the past year, perhaps with the rate of general inflation included, together with estimates of what will be required for the future. It is worthwhile going through the main items of expenditure to check the assumptions used by the accountant are correct for the current situation.

Help the management accountant to understand the way the ward works, the reasons for the grades of staff, types of equipment and procedures. Gather facts. Create an accurate picture of how things function and what they cost. Build up separate accounts for the major functions, move towards resource management even if the computer purchase is still some way off.

The budget is the plan of operation for the year. The expertise of the management accountant should be used to draw the budget up and to find ideas for getting enhanced value for the same expenditure. Be creative. Remember, greater expenditure in one area means a cut in another. Make a list in order of priority for improving patient care and service. Prepare in advance, explore ways to streamline ward stocks of disposables, medicines and stationery. The floor area used for storage uses heat and light. It might be used more productively for another activity. Holding less stocks, perhaps through moving to a 'just-in-time' supplier, could provide extra space. It is important to look at the clinical and management implications of alternative suppliers; the accountant can help with the comparisons.

Read the summaries of the reports from the Audit Commission and the National Audit Office. Their value for money studies provide ideas for improvements. Seek to enhance quality for the same cost.

Watch out for the creeping clinical developments or the empire-builder who rushes into new procedures without counting the cost, expecting staff support without consultation or involvement.

Plan for the whole year. Do not have a 'feast-or-famine' situation from January to March to get back on target. Build in a safety net allocation for each month. Plan that, if unused, the allocation gets carried forward for 2 months and that any remaining in the third month is immediately spent on the piece of equipment, project or course at the top of the ward's list. Make sure it is something that is of benefit to the ward staff in recognition of their part in keeping within the core budget.

Learn about financial management to avoid being blinded by a torrent of figures. Either find a course that gives practical examples or arrange sessions with the local finance officers. Staff can only expect the management accountant to learn about health care if they are willing in turn to learn about the world of health care finance.

Financial support and time to undertake a course may need to be obtained from a senior manager. If a hospital is introducing a new system it has a responsibility to provide staff with the necessary education and training. Devolving budgets requires the same investment in staff. Once personal preparation is complete, arrange for a teaching session on the ward budgets and monthly budget statements. Invite the whole team, clinical and support staff, as their contribution will influence the success of the new system. If at the end of the meeting, the team members cannot make sense of the budget statements to see if the wards are on target or doing better, the management accountant will have to provide a simpler format. It is the financial expert's responsibility to prepare the information so that it is clear and easy to interpret, rather than expect staff to take on trust the expert's interpretation.

Further reading

Department of Health and Social Security (1985) *Health Services Management Budgeting*, HMSO, London.

Darnley, M. (1990) Clinical budgeting – a positive development? *Nursing Standard*, **4**, 15, 37–39.

Darnley, M. (1990) Clinical practice budgeting. *Nursing Standard*, **4**, 46, 47–49.

National Audit Office (1989) *Financial Management in the National Health Service*, HMSO, London.

Or:

National Health Service (1989) *Coronary Heart Disease*, HMSO, London.

Public finance discussion papers, for example:
Roberts, H. (1990) *Outcome and Performance in Health Care,* Discussion
    paper No. 33, Public Finance Foundation, London.

BURNOUT

Burnout is a progressive loss of idealism, energy and purpose,
resulting from stressful work conditions that eventually over-
whelm coping strategies. The only remaining defence is then to
withdraw emotionally from the situation, give up the job or to
give up on the job when:

- empathy turns to apathy;
- involvement to detachment;
- openness to self-protection; and
- trust to suspicion.

Early symptoms of burnout include: overeating; drinking more
alcohol; smoking; and cursing. Tension headaches or other minor
causes of ill health start to increase 'sick' time away from work.
The extra tidying of cupboards or lengthy report-writing take the
individual away from the bedside stress.

Staff appear unfeeling towards patients or staff in their
care; their behaviour may even be callous. The growing sense of
inadequacy and failure is denied. The quality of care is
reduced although techniques and treatments may be carried out
correctly.

Burnout is not just a personal problem, it is an organizational
one. Pushing willing staff too hard to achieve a high-quality
service encourages burnout and then quality falls. Managers also
increase the likelihood of burnout when they seek staff with
noble aspirations and high enthusiasm, knowing inadequate
funding will make it impossible to deliver the professionally
endorsed level of care.

It is very difficult to prevent burnout in hospitals where staff
must work with seriously ill or dying patients. Unresolved
personal feelings and fear of death lead to donning the emotional
armour of detachment. Sending the sufferer on a course or work-
shop, and then returning them to the same stresses, ignores the
cause and allows the manager to rationalize failure to deal with
the problem by blaming the victim.

Unqualified staff can suffer burnout as easily as the professionals. They can feel powerless to influence patient care and treatment. Unfulfilled recruitment promises of training opportunities, unrealistic expectations of job satisfaction and the cynicism of burntout professionals, rub off on the newcomer and permeate the culture. All reduce the quality of the early work experience. The Health Care Assistant programme, with the potential to go on to professional preparation courses, has great potential for reducing such early burnout.

The phenomenon of burnout can be prevented by increasing the support for staff in the workplace. It is part management style and part creating a framework for the more-effective coping strategies, such as talking about work stress, getting advice and taking more control of the decisions that affect daily work. We have emphasized this by writing about **counselling**, **decisions**, the **'honeymoon period'**, **humour**, **promises**, **success** and **vision**. However, the risk of burnout among pathologically conscientious managers is increased by trying to be 'Superman-ager' or 'Superwoman-ager'.

Ward staff face heavy caseloads and a lack of control over the pace of work, if medical staff fail to assess the likely effect of heavy operating lists or heroic treatments. The clinical leaders of the directorate should involve the team in solving the problem and reject the medical staff's defence of 'it's the administrator's problem to find enough staff'. Team decisions share the blame and the praise for success.

Culture shock followed by burnout is likely to increase among *Project 2000*-prepared nurses. The 'tyranny of the should' is intensified by any increase in the gap between theory and the reality of everyday practice. Help should be provided to reduce the fear of not living up to unrealistic standards by developing a framework of preceptorship and setting achievable goals and criteria for measuring these at regular appraisals.

Middle managers have to balance the requirements of those above with those of the staff below. They often feel drowned in the paperwork and struggle along in isolation. Staff appreciate the tough manager who refuses to allow administrators or outsiders to waste staff time. An effective manager aims to be more jealous of the staff's time than of their own while seeing the delegated work is fairly allocated and progress monitored (see Oncken's monkeys in **Delegation**).

The manager should also control personal burnout by arranging regular 'get-togethers' with other managers for mutual support and discussion. This may be through arranging a regular, informal lunch party where each contributes to the food or a buffet before a short evening lecture on a management topic of interest. Managers should only accept realistic objectives for the coming year, while remembering that top managers can experience burnout too. They are often faced with multiple roles, political pressures, a job they were not trained to do and bad publicity if anything in their organization goes wrong.

Further reading

Bond, M. (1986) *Stress and Self-awareness: A Guide for Nurses*. Heinemann, London.

Edelwich, J. and Brodsky, A. (1980) *Burnout: Stages of Disillusionment in the Helping Professions*, Human Sciences Press, London.

Hare, J., Pratt, C.C. and Andrews, D. (1987) Predictors of burnout in professional and paraprofessional nurses working in hospitals and nursing homes. *International Journal of Nursing Studies*, **25**, 2, 105–15.

C

COMMITTEES

Clinical directorates may use committees to involve people from different disciplines to formally agree common action, policies and procedures. Committees keep a formal written record of their deliberations and decisions, the detailed work on items considered by committees having been delegated to small, less-formal working parties. A working party should have a specific purpose and timescale for completion of their work.

Staff time is a resource that should be costed and used with care. Commercial companies, particularly those involved with computer systems, rely on the knowledge and expertise of health care staff in the tailoring of their system to suit a clinical area and can use up a large chunk of staff time. The manager may wish to charge for this time and set it against the cost of the computer system. Managers must also be prepared to pay if they require the skills of others from outside the directorate.

The manager should be assessing the quality of the process followed by an internal committee and examining the output against the investment of time and money. At least once a year each established committee should review its purpose and whether its membership, method of working and frequency of meetings is still appropriate.

There may be opportunities for staff to participate in national or even international committees. This can provide stimulation, raise the profile of the directorate and build a network of useful contacts. Some people become skilled at working through committees to get new ideas adopted or the particular perspectives of a clinical speciality understood and accepted. They may bring back new ideas to share with colleagues as well as collecting opinions to represent the collective expertise of the directorate.

The cost of the staff time involved could be met from the staff-development budget, the advertising budget or as a specific grant from the overall hospital budget.

A committee or working party should consist of people who know the subjects under discussion or can make a constructive contribution. The work of such groups must be monitored to ensure they do not become so specialized that other staff do not understand what they are doing, or that the group members do not spend too long away from the area where they are primarily employed to work. Any reports from such groups should be readable and not have too much money spent on glossy packaging. Before a working party employs outsiders, it should consider whether anyone locally has the desired skills and/or knowledge.

People invited to be part of a committee or working party are expected to do their homework. This involves reading the relevant reports, and, if time is short, at least reading the summary and the parts of the report on which they will be expected to comment. However, short-cuts should not become the 'norm' – often essential information is missed by using 'stop-gap' measures. It is worth writing down anything important one wants to say – just in case it gets forgotten.

Effective committee minutes have an action column that includes the name or initials of the person who is to take the action. Committee members are expected to complete their allocated work before the next meeting or as agreed in the body of the minutes.

Seating arrangements can be important. Occasionally a chairperson will use the seating as a method of control, for example someone who dominates or intimidates during meetings may be allocated a seat out of the direct visual range of the chairperson. A member who feels unfairly manipulated, or who lacks confidence in expressing a point of view, should sit opposite the chairperson.

Repeated destructive or irrelevant comments should be dealt with by the chairperson in private. However, if such behaviour continues, the offender should be censored during the meetings; if this fails then the person should be replaced on the committee.

COMMUNITY HEALTH COUNCIL

The Community Health Council (CHC) draws its members in rotation from local health-related organizations. The wide cross-section can provide a network to link in all their organizations for information exchange and the collection of opinions on the quality of the health service. The CHC can reflect the views of the service users in an anonymous, yet powerful way.

The secretary and chairperson gain much insight into the workings of the local hospitals. Effective ones ensure that their Council acts as a 'ginger' group to help health service staff recognize the changes that the patients and relatives feel would improve the service.

Some health authorities involve the CHC in the purchasing process. A CHC may also work on a broader front with the local authority to influence the provision of both hospital and community care.

Members of the CHC can be invited to join a planning team at the initial stage when policy is being crystallized and also at the design stage they can look at the proposals for action from the consumers' viewpoint.

The secretary of the CHC will also act as 'the patient's friend' in handling a formal complaint. Some CHCs set up their own panel to review the reports on the handling of patient complaints. They may suggest a survey by the CHC to collect opinions from a wider group of patients to establish whether there is a significant problem before meeting hospital or health authority officers to discuss improvements. Regular observation visits with follow-up meetings to discuss the CHCs comments can prove a fruitful source of ideas for improving quality.

The CHC members may be willing to participate with the hospital in surveys that examine the patients' views on the quality of care. Patients may be more open in their comments because they see the CHC as 'on their side'. Since CHC members are volunteers, if they are asked to help a hospital team in this way they should be offered reimbursement of their travel expenses and the secretarial time involved in any collation and analysis.

The Association of Community Health Councils can draw together the best minds from the voluntary sector to examine health care. Their reports provide good ideas for improvements and highlight what the consumer values.

Consider using their patients' charter as a discussion point when developing a philosophy for the ward or directorate.

Further reading

NHS Management Executive (1994) *The operation of Community Health Councils*, EL(94) 4, Department of Health, Leeds.

Association of Community Health Councils for England and Wales (1993) *Performance Standards for CHCs: developing the framework*, ACHEW, 30 Drayton Park, London N5 1PB.

COMPLAINTS

It takes courage and persistence to use the usual hospital complaints process. Value every one that gets through as a golden opportunity to find out more. The ones to worry about are the angry, upset patients or relatives who do not complain to the team but who tell all their family and friends what was wrong.

The *Patient's Charter* sets out the formal rights of complainants in relation to the NHS. These are:

To have any complaint about the NHS services – whoever provides them – investigated and to receive a full and prompt reply from the chief executive or general manager of your hospital. If you are still unhappy, you will be able to take up the case with the Health Service Commissioner. [1]

From April 1993 health authorities and the NHS hospitals had to publish regularly the details of the number of complaints received, and to log how long it took to deal with them.

Obtaining more information on the perceived quality of the service can be very useful. A meeting should be arranged with the complainant, on their territory if possible. If there was a clinical problem the doctor or nurse should be involved, with a second person to act as a witness to what was said. The first meeting is to explore all the 'ins and outs' of the complaint. Notes of the meeting should be recorded. The person dealing with the complaint should avoid sounding defensive, should apologize that there appears to be a problem and promise to look into it straight away. Investigations should start as soon as possible. When staff are interviewed, the manager should also ask for ideas on how the service could be improved.

A second meeting should be arranged to feed back the results. Explain what action has been taken, what further action is planned and confirm it in writing. A note should be made of the deadline set for any further action. Most people realize health service staff are not perfect human beings. All they usually want is an apology and evidence that the staff have taken steps to ensure no one else will suffer the same problem.

The wise manager shares the complaint and findings with the staff involved, with their permission then sharing the situation with the full team. This allows discussion on whether there are further improvements to the quality of the service that could be made.

It is sensible to review each step in the present complaints process as it looks from the patient's point of view. Can it be made easier for a complaint to be made at the time of the problem? Are there leaflets on the formal complaints system for the patient to pick up? Are they friendly in tone? Is the name of the person who should receive the complaint given, or just their job title? Does the leaflet explain the steps that will be followed and the timescale? It is worth reminding the team that an increase in complaints may occur once patients feel the staff care about improving the service. Senior managers sometimes need to be warned to expect this change.

Keep track of all the complaints, review them every quarter for trends. Internal improvements in a ward or department may thwart procedures in other parts of the hospital. A meeting with other managers to seek a solution to a mutual problem may be more effective than the team trying to solve the problem alone.

Some providers of health care services have set up consumer-care departments in order to learn more about the quality of care from complaints, through surveys, and through frequent contact with patients and their families.

Reference

1. Department of Health (1991) *Patient's Charter*, HMSO, London.

Further reading

(1989) Model complaints procedure proposed by CHCs Association, *National Association of Health Authorities News No.133*, **December**, 11.
(1989) *Hospital Complaints Procedure Act 1985 (Commencement) Order*, *Statutory Instrument No 1191*, HMSO, London.

COMPUTERS

Computers are simple machines: they do exactly what they are told to do. The people writing the specification for the system shape it for their own ends. If a manager lets the finance people write the specification for a ward system, the ward staff will become data-entry clerks for the finance team.

A ward-based system must first help the clinical staff by taking out the boring duplication, collecting information and analysing it and by printing out usable, friendly letters and requests. A start may be made by describing a simple system and recording any desirable extensions at appropriate points so that the programmer can write the program to take further sub-routines later on. Some extra points should be included to add in the things everyone forgot.

It is worth spending time with the systems analyst to define and review the present paper systems. Even if it is not included in the computer system, there can be lots to gain from a fresh eye on a familiar path. The analyst can be invited to the clinical area to spend time watching the present system in use. The staff can explain how the wards work, show the layout and talk about the problems created by the present paper work. If the present system does not work well, just transferring it to computer will magnify the problems and produce them at a faster rate.

It is unnecessary to learn how to program a computer and it can be addictive. The wise manager learns enough to be able to be able to spot when the technicians are trying to hide behind the jargon, to know what is really possible and to state the clinical and managerial requirements in clear terms. Confidence in using a computer will be helpful.

Computers can process a mass of data and a manager may be tempted to ask for all the possible permutations to be produced. Quality will be enhanced by being clear how the information will be used. The action to be taken on each report should be described in writing. Where there will be no opportunity to use a report then it is not worth requesting its production. The collection of data and the production of reports takes time and therefore uses resources.

Be prepared to take risks. While a computer can attach an electronic personal identification tag to every entry, it is rare that it will be needed. Every tag takes up space. Computer memory costs money. Statistically the risk of litigation over one item of care is very slight. Instead, limit the number of people who can make or change entries.

A staff training programme should be provided to give every-one who will use the keyboard enough time to 'get to grips' with it. Dummy records and data should also be available at the ward terminals so staff can practise with all the usual background distractions. The quality of work achieved will be related to the amount of practice achieved just before the system 'goes live'.

Be aware that general managers tend to underestimate the budget required for the whole programme. As training comes near the end, if it goes over budget there will be a temptation to cut the funds for training. If staff cannot achieve confidence and mastery at the start, it may be months or years before they do – and what happens to the quality until they get it?

When the system is ready for use, run the manual and the computer system in tandem. Do not stop the manual system until the team feel happy the computer system is working properly. If necessary buy in extra staff time to cope with the overlap. Use the costs to press the computer people to put matters right.

Remember to register the data collected, together with the intended uses, with the Data Protection Registrar. Patients have a right to a copy of any personal data kept on computer; a procedure for its release should be available.

Further reading

Burnard, P. (1990) So you think you need a computer? *Professional Nurse,* **6**, 2, 119–20.

Code, H. (1987) Forty days to find the data. *Health Service Journal,* **97** (5061), **July 30**, 880.

Kinn, S. and Siann, T. (1993) *Computers and Medical Audit,* Chapman & Hall, London.

Tilson, S. (1987) Data Protection: Unleashing access to information. *Health Service Journal,* 97 (5061), **July 30**, 878.

Tongue, C. (1987) Data protection: keeping out the prying eyes. *Health Service Journal,* 97 (5061), **July 30**, 879–80.

CONFLICT

Open disagreement between a manager and staff or among staff is healthy, provided that it is kept low key in public. The manager should be aware that there are people who thrive on conflict and may consciously, or unconsciously, try to create it rather than solve problems.

Conflict can be creative but needs careful handling when discussing underlying beliefs and values about health care. When the same vision is shared, the conflict then lies in the route and speed of travel to achieve the agreed level of quality.

When called upon to solve a problem rooted in conflicting viewpoints, avoid compromise as neither side will be satisfied and the manager then becomes part of their problem. Choose one side or the other. Make it clear that the winner takes full responsibility for making the idea work, and that good points from rival ideas can be incorporated only if the winner chooses to do so, and without further discussion. In this way the person who must win every battle, on or off the field, can be controlled by the manager. Discuss with the looser the reason why your decision went against them. Set a date to evaluate the outcome.

CONTACTS

A manager should get to know other ward managers, teachers and researchers with an interest in the same field. Pioneering can be a lonely business. A chat over the 'phone or a monthly meeting can provide a safety valve and new ideas to solve a worrying, knotty problem.

A network of like-minded people may cover a large area. When the nursing process was beginning to be introduced to wards, the pioneering days were so tough, folk spent much of the day travelling in their own time to attend a 2-hour meeting for support from colleagues. Once the changes became accepted practice, so the need for membership of the group evaporated. Meanwhile, those new to the role of change agent or starting to introduce the system began to join the group.

CONTINUING EDUCATION DEPARTMENT

The manager should consider if the local continuing education department is providing the directorate with the education and training of the required quality. It is sensible to obtain a copy of the department's prospectus of courses and compare the content and costs with others that are offering the same services. Consider the cost of staff travelling to other areas and the advantages of the familiar environment. Most local teaching staff are pleased to help and advise clinical staff. If there is any uncertainty about the suitability of a course, evaluations from an earlier group can be requested. However, if the department cannot provide what is required, then take the business elsewhere.

The directorate's share of the continuing education and training budget should be examined to see if there is a need to invest more to improve the amount or quality of education. Individual performance reviews linked to staff development enables the educational needs to be identified and allows clear goals to be set. Proposed new activities may require a preparatory programme of advanced professional education. Such changes should be built into the directorate's strategy and budget.

The educators should be told of the directorate's long-term plans for staff development so they can take these into account in their strategy. Regional manpower plans may influence the availability of courses. When staff have attended external courses their evaluation and comments should be fed back to the course organizer.

It is good practice to agree the expected outcomes from staff members who are to attend continuing-education sessions. On completion and, after a set period back at work, these can be used to mutually assess the effect of the course. The educators should be given a copy of such assessments so that a partnership develops between them and the clinical staff.

There are increasing opportunities in open and distance learning for staff unable to travel to external courses. The manager can demonstrate a commitment to improving the quality of the experience by facilitating the development of a local support group which purchases materials or loans books, agreeing set time off for study or arranging relevant clinical visits.

Further reading

Bailey, D. (1990) Open learning: the role of the tutor. *Nursing Times*, **86**, 47, 46–48.

Department of Health (1989) *A Strategy for Nursing*, Department of Health, London.

English National Board (1989) *Regulations and Guidelines for the Approval of Institutions and Courses*, English National Board, London.

Swaffield, L. (1990) Open learning, no through road. *Nursing Times*, **86**, 47, 44–45.

UKCC (1993) Post-Registration Education and Practice: Proposed standards and principles for education, Annex 2 for Registrar's Letter

8/93, UK Central Council for Nursing, Midwifery and Health Visiting, London.

Wright, S. (1992) Continuing education, who meets the cost? *Nursing Standard*, 6, **16**, 34–35.

Wright, S. and Ashton, F. (1992) Training-and-development. *Nursing Standard*, **6**, 45, 50–51.

CONTROL – QUALITY OF EQUIPMENT

Equipment and disposables must be safe to use, must do the job required with the minimum of effort and be effective. Small teams of users can be set up to prepare specifications of the 'must do. . .,' the 'must last . . .,' 'helpful if it could do . . .'. Ask the team to circulate their draft specification to all the other users. Give a deadline of 5 working days for comments.

The team then revises the specification and asks the supplies staff to prepare a list of products and prices that meets it. The supplies department should be asked to obtain the published research data to check the claims made in the manufacturer's advertisements.

The Department of Health spend large amounts of money on testing mechanical and other equipment only for their reports to disappear into supplies departments. The wise manager requests a copy of such reports before making the final selection.

Test the two cheapest products to confirm that they match the specification. If they match, add them to the approved list and ban new purchases of all other forms of that type of equip-ment. Arrange any staff training in the use and care of the equipment as part of the purchasing package. Request an extra set of the user notes or manual for the reference section of the library.

Bold commercial representatives can be sent direct to the supplies officer for the specification data, particularly if they try to creep into the wards to try to market their product directly to the staff.

Consider attaching a monitoring card to each CSSD (Central Sterile Supply Unit)/(Theatre Sterile Supply Unit) TSSU proce-dure pack. For example, on a catheterization pack request on the label information on:

- date of use;
- job title of person setting out the equipment;
- job title of person inserting the catheter;

- size and type of catheter used;
- reason for catheterization.

Follow-up by monitoring the date and nature of any urinary infection or mechanical problems with the catheter. Cost any antibiotics required and so on. Use the data to look for trends such as infections linked to the staff carrying out the procedure or problems from a particular size of catheter. Use the information in quality meetings to explore how the equipment is contributing to reduced quality for patients.

Further reading

Department of Health: Health Notices – various; Health Technical memoranda – various.

CONTROL – QUALITY OF STAFF

Quality control starts at the beginning; therefore new team members should be chosen carefully. An allowance should be made for culture shock in staff from other countries and those who are returning to work after several years.

A core staff-orientation plan should be devised. The core programme should include visits and time spent observing or working in any department where the directorate has special link-relationships. Clinical staff may need updating in some clinical procedures. Involvement in the regular fire lectures and cardiac resuscitation programmes should be arranged.

Consideration should be given to the type of skills the new person will require to enable them to give a quality performance. The manager should consult with the person who is to be orientated and the team member who will act as preceptor. Perspectives may differ. A review of the important contacts with support services and those involved in direct patient care will ensure that new staff do not have to spend time meeting people that they are not likely to see or speak to ever again. The core staff-orientation plan can then be adapted to suit the individual needs of the new person.

At the end of the first week the manager should spend some time with the new staff member, evaluating the effectiveness of the programme. Changes and additions can then be made to the programme for the succeeding weeks.

Nurses who have had a significant break in their career will need to attend a 'back to nursing' course. They will also need to work with a more senior experienced nurse who can act as a preceptor [2]. The new member of staff should not be left in charge of a ward or department until the manager is confident that the quality of work and judgement is up to the required standard for the directorate.

Quality control can be carried out formally through the performance-review process; clear objectives should be agreed and then used at the next review to assess progress. A career-development plan should also be compiled. The objectives should be realistic, for if they are not discontent or burnout can occur.

Informal quality control comes through monitoring current performance and the discussion of problems and solutions. Praise should be given for effort or a task completed well. Censorious action should not be carried out publicly unless there is a risk to the safety of the patients or to staff.

Where the performance of an individual member of staff is less than satisfactory, it may be necessary to hold a formal meeting. This should be conducted in private with objectives for improvement and a plan for the additional help that may be required. A date should be set to review formally the level of improvement that has to be demonstrated. A detailed note should be placed in the personnel file with a copy to the individual. Such formal action may become the first step in a disciplinary process.

In 1992, all barriers to trade between countries covered by the *Single European Act, 1987* were removed to give a single unified market. The free movement of nationals within these countries should lead to the establishment of equal standards in education and training in health care. The EEC has been involved with nurse education since 1979 and changes in the time-allocation to components of the curriculum were made. However, the EEC has no jurisdiction over daily nursing practice or other aspects of health care delivery [1]. The directorate may wish to consider staff-exchange schemes and offering language classes as part of a wider programme of development.

Reference

1. Trevelyan, J. (1990) 1992 and all that. *Nursing Times,* **86**, 12, 225–227.

2. UKCC (1993) Post Registration Education and Practice: Annex to Registrar's Letter 1/93. United Kingdom Central Council for Nursing, Midwifery and Health Visiting, London.

Further reading

Office of Health Economics (1988) *Health Service in Europe. Briefing No. 24*, Office of Health Economics, London.

COUNSELLING

Counselling is not discipline with kid gloves on! At its simplest it is listening, reflecting back what is said, and supporting the individual in solving a work-related problem. The individual may seek someone to give counsel, or the manager may feel action is needed to help a member of staff to work through a problem. It follows only after education and coaching have failed to achieve the required improvement in performance. Counselling seeks to enable the individual to chose and to make the changes.

Preparation for the counsellor requires thinking through the key issues and identifying the changes in behaviour that will be required. A time and venue should be chosen that will help reduce stress from the situation. It is cruel to expect people to wait for days worrying about what is going to be said. It is considerate, for example, to arrange in the morning to meet in a quiet office in the afternoon.

At a counselling session, the manager should state the problem and ask the individual to comment. The manager should listen, reflecting on whether personal management style has contributed to the problem. The individual's explanation and any intended behaviour change should be reflected back and gently explored. The decision on action should be made by the individual, not the manager. A date to review progress may be agreed. It should not be changed by the manager without a very good reason.

A deep-seated personal problem requires great skill and training to help the individual review personal matters and to make decisions. Work problems often involve home and family. It needs time, quiet and privacy. It needs to be separate from work relationships. It is wiser to find a fully qualified counsellor to help with such problems, as the role of manager can inter-fere with the role of counsellor in such situations. Check the counsellor also has a confidential support system to prevent over-involvement.

Forward-looking hospitals provide a referral service through the confidential occupational health scheme. Some will subsidize the cost of counselling sessions. Others provide referral but the member of staff has to foot the bill. The individual member of staff must seek the help. Counsellors will not accept someone 'sent' by a manager. Health care staff can be very hard judges of their own performance. Counselling may be helpful when those used to success are suddenly hit by failure.

A self-help group for staff to discuss any work-related problems that are causing them stress may arise from meetings to discuss ethical issues in a ward. In high-stress areas or sites undergoing a period of rapid change, it may be helpful to arrange for an outside counsellor to attend a group meeting of the staff without a manager present. It may take several sessions before the staff feel able to reveal the depth of their distress.

All health care professionals need some counselling skills to enable them to help patients in a positive and therapeutic way. The skills include [1]:

- listening and attending;
- using open questions;
- reflecting content and feelings;
- summarizing;
- checking and understanding.

Acquiring such skills does not make an individual a fully trained counsellor.

Reference

1. Burnard, P. (1991) Acquiring minimal counselling skills: clinical counselling. *Nursing Times*, **5**, 46, 37–39.

Further reading

BAC, *BAC Training Directory*, British Association of Counselling, 37 Sheep Street, Rugby.

Burnard, P. (1989) *Counselling Skills for Professionals*, Chapman & Hall, London.

Macleod Clark, J., Hopper, L. and Jesson, A. (1991) Communication skills, progress to counselling. *Nursing Times*, **87**, 8, 41–43.
Murgatroyd, S. (1986) *Counselling and Helping*, Methuen, London.

CREDIT

The world often seems to be divided into those who produce the results and those who get the credit. Ways to ensure the directorate, team or member of the staff get the credit include:

- having a team logo sticker, which is then used on all publications, however humble;
- organizing an open day or seminars to describe the results;
- asking the staff to make the presentation to senior managers on their work;
- nominating staff for external awards;
- starting internal awards, within the directorate or hospital, for improved quality;
- announcing achievements in the hospital newsletter;
- including public thanks during meetings and presentations;
- noting the successful completion of a project in the personal records of the participants and mentioning it in any subsequent job references;
- putting the staff member as the first name on the list of authors in a journal article;
- listing the names of members of the working group on patient-information leaflets;
- inviting all the staff to the launch party and including their names in the related press release.

D

DECISIONS

Keep these as low down in the team hierarchy as possible. Time is precious. There are two kinds of decisions: those that put life and health at risk and those that do not. If the first kind go wrong they are expensive in the time required to correct the situation and sometimes in litigation. They also create tension and worry for the staff. It should be made clear which decisions can only be taken by the manager.

It can be helpful to develop the habit of reviewing the contents of the manager's in-tray for work where the decisions can be delegated to other members of the team. They may be better placed to draw up the plan of action. Capitalize on the talent of the team. The power to make decisions increases job satisfaction.

Discuss and get advice from the specialists if the decision will have a knock-on effect on the budget, or on how other departments work. Consider what additional resources may be needed in order that the decision will be taken with confidence. Set the parameters, then delegate.

If staff make a mistake, focus on what has been learnt and done to correct it. The manager should consider whether the right level of support and monitoring was provided (the insurance policy for that particular monkey, see page 39).

If the staff are unused to such power, coaching will help develop decision-making skills. The manager may consider working out, with the staff, lists of the steps to be used. The manager must keep a discreet watch for indicators of potential problems such as procrastination, shifting of responsibility or a selective search for information to bolster the reasons for inaction. Staff who become hypervigilant and seek a mass of information are showing mental conflict and need help from the manager to clarify their difficulties.

Group decisions that bolster the leader's view are not confined to tyrannies. The strong team spirit of an isolated group, unused to methodically seeking evidence and with a low self-esteem, will agree with the leader in the face of objective evidence that the decision is wrong. The dissenter is out, so self-censorship comes in. Conviction is all and, as failure is unthinkable, the contingency plans are never laid.

Group-think is death to excellence. The wise manager treasures the dissenter.

Further reading

Jansis, I.L. and Mann, L. (1977) *Decision Making*, The Free Press, London.

DELEGATION

The ability to delegate is a necessary attribute for all managers. Quality is everybody's business. Pick the member of the team for whom the experience will mean the most for professional development of personal growth. Consider if coaching will be necessary.

A description of the framework within which the member of staff must work should be provided. It should make clear which decisions can be made without reference back to the manager. Delegation involves the team member in taking on extra responsibilities.

At the first sign of overspending, managers should not introduce tight control by requiring senior people to endorse every requisition for supplies. Instead, the manager should go through the problem with the staff who normally do the ordering, and together plan how to tackle it. Delegating responsibility for ordering stores to an agreed stock level to the ward clerks can be very cost-effective and free the time of the clinical staff for their clinical work.

The manager who feels harassed by frequent requests for decisions or help with problems from staff, should remember Oncken's monkeys [1]. He suggests that a 'monkey' is the next move in a process. As soon as the manager offers help with a problem that next move (or monkey) transfers to the manager and needs action (or feeding). Promise a progress report on the problem and the manager becomes the worker, and the member of staff the boss. The wise manager does not pick up other people monkeys but becomes proactive rather than reactive.

The harassed manager has to learn to recognize which monkeys belong to the role, handing the rest back to the appropriate member of staff, with an apology for the delay as well as instructions for the action programme to be followed (care and feeding). The manager should describe the next move, use action words such as: prepare, give, get, formulate options or recommendations and encouraging the new owner of the monkey (next move) to break the required sequence of action into small steps (bite-size pieces).

Quality development programmes can create many 'monkeys' for the unwary manager. Some activities may no longer be necessary, so that particular monkey can be killed off or stopped. The staff may be able to share the burden by carrying some of the manager's monkeys for a while, leaving only those that only the manager can handle.

Oncken suggests that the manager should insure against expensive mistakes by either requesting that the new owner seeks approval for a proposed action, or by acting and then informing the manager. He also suggests arranging a regular check-up date to confirm progress and spot problems. This way a 'monkey' will not starve to death from lack of attention (attention and feeding).

Reference

1. Blanchard, K., Oncken, W. and Burrows, H. (1990) *The One Minute Manager Meets the Monkey*, Collins, London.

Further reading

Holroyd, G. (1976) *How to Delegate: A Practical Guide*, Mantec, Rugby.

DISOBEDIENCE

A commander-in-chief (manager) cannot take as an excuse for his mistakes in warfare (management) an order given by his minister (director) or his sovereign (general manager), when the person giving the order is absent from the field of operations and is imperfectly aware or wholly unaware of the latest state of affairs. It follows that any commander-in-chief (manager) who undertakes to carry out a plan that he/she considers defective is at fault; he/she must put forward his/her reasons, insist on the plan being changed, and finally tender his/her resignation rather than be the instrument of his army's (team's) downfall.

(Based on Napoleon's *Military Maxims and Thoughts*.)

E

EDUCATING FOR QUALITY

A sound educational programme is essential when implementing quality assurance initiatives effectively. The manager of the directorate should consult with senior managers to discuss the breadth and depth of the hospital-wide programme, so that the directorate and ward initiatives do not duplicate effort.

Initially, education should be targeted at the co-ordinator and/or facilitator of any quality assurance initiatives. If standard setting is to be undertaken, the leader of each group should be included.

The facilitators need a firm knowledge base and a commitment to total quality management. It is important that they have inter-personal skills that will enable them to support, teach and advise others. According to Kemp and Richardson [1], they also need some experience of the theory and practice of teaching. Look at what other directorates are doing for quality facilitators. If there is nothing available, consider joining forces to organize a work-shop, if necessary employing an outside consultant to assist. Facilitation requires time and it may be difficult to add the role to a heavy workload. The manager may act in a co-ordinating role to any quality assurance group within the wards of the direc-torate.

This will include:

- identifying the needs of the group;
- providing the resources to carry out the work;
- choosing the group leader;
- co-ordinating and monitoring the work of one or more groups.

The role of the leader of a standard setting group should be taken by someone with a sound knowledge of the subject to be evalu-ated, good interpersonal skills, some administrative talent and a firm commitment to evaluate and improve practice. The role will include chairing the group.

All staff involved in quality assurance initiatives need:

- an introduction to the concepts and methods of any quality assurance monitoring system being used;
- an understanding of the terminology and the data-collecting procedure;
- an understanding of how to respond to the results.

The education and information can be given at a study day, ideally away from the wards. Such days include time to examine the proposed quality monitoring tool and a question-and-answer session. A short handout summarizing key points from the presentation can be helpful. A glossary of terms and a bibliography may also be provided.

If it is intended to buy in a monitoring system, a representative from the firm could be invited to describe the system; there may, however, be a charge for this.

The quality monitors/observers/raters/auditors need the same preparation, as well as practice in collecting and collating data in an environment where mistakes can be made without embarrassment. Preparation for later inter-observer reliability testing is necessary, followed by a trial of the monitoring tool, preferably in a similar area to the ward or directorate. This should be followed by a final time for review and discussion.

Inter-observer reliability testing means achieving a high level of agreement among observers using the same tool. Calculate the percentage of time that two or more observers, independently collecting information from the same source at the same time, agree on what was observed. The workshop for this activity involves participants recapping information about the tool and then practising, for example with a video of a clinical situation, so that written observations can be compared and discussed. Exploring the different interpretations helps to develop a consensus view of the key components represented by each score. The practice sessions may need to be repeated several times. If inter-observer reliability is poor, the tool must be revised or discarded.

To set standards, the staff involved need education in the following:

- information about measurement;
- how to set standards and criteria;
- group dynamics.

Practice should be given in writing standards and criteria for later discussion by the group.

When planning any educational exercise, the manager should state the aim, consider the cost and, if necessary, seek advice from teaching staff as to the best methods to use. Consultation with the staff who will be involved, to enable them to voice any fears and concerns, is time well spent if notice is taken of their views and suggestions. A strategy, with objectives, should be written for each session and a review carried out after the session to assess the outcomes and quality of the education and also the manager's own action.

Reference

1. Kemp, N. and Richardson, E. (1990) *Quality Assurance in Nursing Practice*, Butterworth Heinemann, Oxford.

Further reading

Ellis, R. (ed.) (1989). *Professional Competencies and Quality Assurance in the Caring Professions*, Chapman & Hall, London.
Griffiths, W. (1986) Action learning for quality assurance – a diary. *International Journal of Health Care and Quality Assurance*, 1, 1, 29–31.
Haussman, R.K.B. and Hegyvary, S.T. (1976) Field testing: the nursing quality monitoring methodology. *Nursing Research*, 25, 5, 324–31.
NHS Management Executive (1991), *Measuring The Quality*, teaching notes, NHS Management Executive, Quarry House, Quarry Hill, Leeds, LS2 7UE.
Sale, D. (1988) Down Dorset way. *Nursing Times*, 13, 84, 28, 31–33.
Satow, A. and Evans, M. (1983) *Working with groups*, HES/TACADE, 2 Mount Street, Manchester, M25 NG.
World Health Organization (1986) Nursing/Midwifery in Europe: Quality Assurance. *Nursing Unit Information Bulletin*, 3, 1. (Regional Office Nursing Unit, WHO Regional Office for Europe, 8 Scherfigsverj, DK-2100, Copenhagen.)

EDUCATION IN CLINICAL AREAS

Each directorate should have an education and training component within its strategy. All members of the staff have a right to continuing education and training. The increasing speed of change in knowledge makes it essential if the quality of care in the performance of their duties is to keep up with the expectations of the public. Several of the health care professions now require evidence of such updating for confirmation of permission to practice. For example, nurses are expected to comply with the guidelines of the UK Central Council's (1990) post-registration education and practice project (PREPP) [1]. This emphasizes self-development, from exploring personal clinical practice in some depth as well as taught material.

In order to influence quality the manager needs to create an effective learning environment. To do this it is necessary to:

- foster a forward-looking approach by implementing research-based practice;
- remain aware of professional developments;
- keep up with the changes in the students' curricula;
- foster good relationships between teachers and staff;
- remain aware of the range of education facilities available;
- enable staff to undertake further education.

An effective learning environment is one where staff feel supported and where stress levels are controlled so that staff are not in poor health or too tired to concentrate.

There are times when the manager may wish to formalize learning within the clinical area. A variety of teaching methods can be used including:

- the seminar where the group and the teacher discuss a specific topic;
- tutorials on a one-to-one or small-group basis;
- practical demonstrations; followed by supervised practice;
- role play.

Experiential learning can be a powerful approach to exploring the quality of the environment provided for those with sensory deficits. For example, a member of staff is asked to identify with a deaf person by using earplugs while spending time undertaking the same activities experienced by a patient. The example is also helpful where quality is to be monitored by interviews. The experience and ideas arising from it can then be related to the other members of the ward or quality assurance team.

Before sending a member of staff on a course, the manager needs to consider the desired benefits to the person and the hospital. Questions to be considered include whether the person has the necessary background and ability to benefit. The pre-course requirements and objectives should be reviewed. It can be wasteful to send someone to a course that covers skills or knowledge they have already acquired. Although a course is not an effective way to cope with burnout, someone who lacks motivation may be stimulated by material that builds on existing skills and explores a wider context for using them. Part-time staff should be given the same opportunities to attend educational activities as the full-time people.

An alternative to a course may be distance learning. The choice is not to be taken lightly as it requires motivation to complete the work. Educationalists will be able to advise on the best packages available.

Quality can be increased by the application of knowledge. Staff cannot use knowledge they do not have. The speed of expansion of the range and depth of knowledge about health care is now so rapid that the manager has to ensure easy access to new material. Libraries are changing their function from being book stores to access points to a range of materials, including videos, compact discs, computer-held lists of abstracts and databases as well as bulletin boards and electronic information exchanges. The librarian should be able to provide lists of new material relevant to specified topics of use to the directorate.

Some staff have a natural flair for and are interested in teaching. The manager should help develop such talent through relevant courses and by providing opportunities to teach others. It is expected that where a ward accepts student nurses for clinical placements, the staff nurses will attend mentorship courses. Sisters and charge nurses should attend a teaching and assessment course such as the English National Board course 997/998, which focuses on clinical practice. The City and Guilds 7305 further and adult education teachers' certificate course should also be considered, particularly for those in non-clinical roles. It is worth noting that teaching skills are transferable to other settings such as presenting information at meetings. Effective teaching during patient-education sessions and in explaining new techniques can improve the overall performance quality of the ward or directorate.

It is sensible for the manager to identify a member of staff to oversee and organize teaching sessions for ward staff. These sessions may be shared between wards. The manager should request a draft plan of the study sessions. Students and new staff can be involved in presenting part of the material – this is a good way for them to learn. Time needs to be set aside for preparation. The manager should provide sufficient resources, for example, a portable overhead projector. One of the educational staff may be prepared to give a small demonstration on how to use visual aids effectively.

When seminars or tutorials are to be given, they should be held in a room kept at a comfortable temperature and free of non-essential interruptions. The teaching programme should be circulated and the night staff given the opportunity to attend or to have a repeat session held especially for them.

The teaching programme, teaching notes and visual aids may provide a teaching package of use to other wards or directorates. This should be tested to confirm it has a wider application and is effective. It may be appropriate to seek help in marketing it; the money raised can be used by the directorate for further educational activities or resources.

Reference

1. UK Central Council for Nursing, Midwifery and Health Visiting (1993) *Post-registration Education and Practice: Proposed Standards and Principles for Education.* Annex 2 to Registrar's Letter 8.93, UKCC, London.

Further reading

Bailey, D. (1990) Open learning: the role of the tutor. *Nursing Times,* **86**, 47, 46–48.
Barnett, D.E. (1974) Ward teaching. *Nursing Times,* **70** (27) **July 4**, 1046–47.
Fretwell, J. (1982) *Ward Teaching and Learning: Sister and the Learning Environment,* Royal College of Nursing, London.
Reid, N G. (1985) *Wards in Chancery?* Royal College of Nursing, London.
RCN (1985) *Commission on Nursing Education – The Education of Nurses: A New Dispensation,* (Judge Report), Royal College of Nursing, London.

EGO MASSAGE

A major effort to survey all the wards, feed the data into a computer and then distribute the report with many statistics, 3 months too late for effective action is just ego massage for managers!

Avoid it at all costs. If there is no promise to make changes based on the results – do not start the survey.

Uninformed use of information technology, such as computers, because it seems the modern thing to do will reduce the credibility of the manager and, by diverting resources, risk a negative effect on quality. It is more effective to have a series of short, tightly focused surveys, with action taken on the results before the next one starts.

EQUIPMENT

The quality of all equipment must be fit for the purpose and tested before purchase and during the initial period of use. It should also be checked on a regular, planned basis. The *Health and Safety at Work Act 1974* also requires that staff should use equipment correctly.

As part of the purchase order, the supplier can be required to provide teaching sessions for staff and literature prior to the introduction of any new item, particularly monitoring equipment. A file of technical information for easy reference should be compiled. The recall and understanding of the use and care of the equipment can be tested with a quiz. This is of particular importance if the item is rarely used but may contribute to the resuscitation of an ill patient. A weekend quiz during a 'quiet' shift with a small prize, such as a chocolate bar, can increase motivation. The night staff must not be forgotten in the instruction and testing programme.

The 'control of infection team' should be consulted about the cleaning of new equipment during use and prior to inspection, service or repair. The works department may need to use special equipment or procedures where sealed units cannot be decontaminated on the ward. Advice can be sought from the health and safety officer or the occupational health department. The quality of protection from the risk of infection provided for both staff and patients should be checked at intervals, together with observations to establish if the policies are being followed.

Special cleaning equipment may be required to render everyday equipment free of pathogenic bacteria. For example, a long 'bottle-brush' for cleaning inside the tubing into which the seat of a portable bathing hoist should slot [1].

Research reports on the control of infection have shown that some procedures are worthless rituals, such as wearing overshoes in theatre, whereas common items, such as worn, torn mattresses are definite sources of infection [2]. A regular news sheet giving the reasons for change may be circulated so that all the team members understand the reasons for the change.

Where emergency equipment is used infrequently, provide a 'simple guide' listing all the steps required to set it up and turn it on. Attach the guide to the equipment. Photographs can be helpful. Timed practice runs with an award for the fastest time can be fun and improve skills. A programme of regular updating and practice at using cardiopulmonary resuscitation equipment should be held for all staff.

Quality in practice

In a maternity unit, one source of friction between a delivery suite and the neonatal intensive care unit came from requests for help to set up the mobile incubator with ventilator. It took several steps to set it up for use. The staff of the neonatal unit had held several teaching sessions for their colleagues but in the heat of an emergency the labour ward staff still rang the unit for urgent advice. A checklist attached to the machine solved the problem overnight.

References

1. Murdoch, S. (1986) Hazards in hoists. *Nursing Times*, **86**, 49, 68 and 70.
2. Loomes, S. (1988) Is it safe to lie down in hospital? *Nursing Times*, **84**, 49, 63–65.

Further reading

Department of Health (London) circulars and booklets: *'Decontamination of Health Care Equipment Prior to Inspection, Service or Repair'*; Health Equipment Notices; Health Technical Memoranda.

ETHICS

Ethics involve autonomy and rights, and their effect on the quality of life of the individual and society as a whole. One person's rights can imply another person's duties, and therefore accountability and responsibility [1].

The components involve the ability to reason, to have a choice and freedom to make it, the ability to act and to consider the impact of such action. The degree to which these are present for the patient, and their interaction, create the complexity in identifying the ethically acceptable approach to care and treatment. Medical ethics are of increasing public interest as the limitations on choice of treatment grow with the reduction in available resources to meet the competing needs of the population.

Ethical issues which impinge on the quality of care include:

- respect for life;
- informed consent;
- personal freedom;
- the patient's right to be involved in decisions about care and treatment;
- new treatments;
- maintaining dignity and choice;
- privacy and confidentiality.

Everyday work with patients will touch on many of these issues. Unless there are clear guidelines and the beliefs and values of the hospital are clearly stated, each person giving care must analyse each problem afresh and find a solution from their own value system. This may lead to uneven quality in the delivery of patient care.

Ethical problems can result in litigation. The increasing interest in medical law has resulted in a range of books and pamphlets.

The law has been used to state the rules governing specific practices, for example, conscientious objection to abortion, contraceptive advice to minors and embryo research.

Patients and staff, purchasers and providers have to operate in a climate of mutual trust and understanding. Each party expects the other to act ethically, taking into account the needs and interests of the other.

District health authorities were required to have an ethics committee. Until recently much of their work had concerned research proposals; now they are beginning to be asked to advise on other issues. Health care providers have also set up their own ethics committees. The commercial pressures and the introduction of the business experiences of non-executive directors in the early 1990s created tensions with the established public-sector ethos.

Detailed guidelines became necessary to set out clear standards of conduct.

On clinical research the EC guidance is likely to become a directive eventually. It includes quality assurance to verify data and an audit by the sponsor of the research [2, 3].

Quality assurance activities may require ethics committee approval. Managers should submit any questionnaire or survey form with the protocol to the chairman for advice. Permission may be given under 'Chairman's action' and reported to the full committee. All research proposals should be submitted well before the proposed starting date.

Consideration should also be given as to whether there are ethical issues regularly raised by the specific work of the wards. The advice of the ethics committee may be helpful to the staff.

Professional practice is influenced by statutory and professional bodies. The UK Central Council for Nursing, Midwifery and Health Visiting (UKCC) has a standards and ethics committee and has joined with the General Medical Council to discuss subjects of mutual interest [4]. The Royal Colleges and unions also provide advice to their members.

Nursing and midwifery staff have a responsibility to report any potential or actual problems, for example, inadequate staffing levels, that put patients at risk. This is covered by points 10 and 11 of the UKCC [5] Code of Conduct.

The UKCC guidelines can be of use to other disciplines [6]. They have covered autonomous HIV testing, fetal technology, exercising accountability, advertising and commercial sponsorship.

When resources are stretched there is a temptation to seek sponsorship for new projects. However, acceptance of such sponsorship should not carry any obligations. A small plaque or acknowledgement to record the generosity of the benefactor may be acceptable. Large advertisements, use of a company logo on uniforms, or an agreement to push a specific product such as stoma equipment are not! Staff must exercise caution over the 'drug company lunches', free gifts, sponsorships and fellowships.

The manager can help staff fulfil their personal responsibility for maintaining high standards of behaviour and practice by:

• debating beliefs about patient care, autonomy and responsibility;

- maintaining a file of recent journal articles on relevant ethical issues;
- raising ethical issues for discussion in ward meetings;
- developing a procedure that allows staff to obtain advice on ethical dilemmas facing them in their daily practice and to record a conscientious objection to participating in specific practices, for example, electroconvulsive therapy.

References

1. Chapman, C. (1980) The rights and responsibilities of nurses and patients. *Journal of Advanced Nursing* , **5**, 127–34.
2. Bull, M. (1989) Making ethical committees effective. *Bulletin of Medical Ethics*, **53**, 13–17.
3. (1989) European guidance on medical research. *Bulletin of Medical Ethics*, **56**, 8–10.
4. UKCC (1989) The Standards and Ethics Committee – looking back and looking forward. *Register No. 7*, UK Council for Nursing, Midwifery and Health Visiting, London.
5. UKCC (1993) *Code of Professional Conduct for the Nurse, Midwife and Health Visitor*. 3rd edn., UK Central Council for Nursing, Midwifery and Health Visiting, London.
6. UKCC (1989) *Exercising Accountability – A Framework to Assist Nurses, Midwives and Health Visitors to Consider Ethical Aspects of Professional Practice*, UK Central Council for Nursing, Midwifery and Health Visiting, London.

Further reading

Brazier, M. (1987) *Medicine, Patients and the Law*, Penguin, London.
Ginzer, M., Davies, J., McPherson, K. and Black, N. (1990) Ethics committees and health service research. *Journal of Public Health Medicine*, **12**, 3–4, 190–96.
Phillips, M. and Dawson, J. (1985) *Doctors' Dilemmas: Medical Ethics and Contemporary Science*, Harvester Wheatsheaf, London.
Thompson, I.E., Melia, K.M. and Boyd K.M. (1989) *Nursing Ethics*, Churchill Livingstone, Edinburgh.
Tschudin, V. (1986) *Ethics in Nursing: The Caring Relationship*, Heinemann, London.

EXCELLENCE

Excellence is to surpass others in one or more qualities. It takes considerable energy, flexibility and commitment.

The 1980s saw senior managers urged to introduce self-improvement programmes into their organizations and 'to do more with less'. Commercial firms used excellence to gain a competitive edge over rivals. Once most of the others caught up, the customer regained a wider choice of firms from which to buy. Health services in the UK are continuing to face these challenges in the 1990s. NHS and private health care providers have to develop centres of excellence for the treatment of specific diseases.

Excellence has a cost. Essentially it is attention to detail and this requires sufficient time, staff and equipment. In many areas, an effective and efficient service may be all that is required. For many years the difference between private and NHS health care has rested on the excellence of the hotel-type services and the opportunity to choose the medical attendant and date of admission, rather than on the overall medical and nursing treatment. The NHS is now paying more attention to patient preferences and improving the quality of hotel services.

The manager must be clear about the cost of achieving excellence in each new area of activity. Unless it is possible to use resources in such a way as to do more work with less, it may be necessary to do less or nothing in one area in order to excel in the new area. It is important that the manager recognizes what cannot be done well.

The clinical team may have to assess the level of performance being achieved in the unusual surgical operations, or medical illness. Work on the 'Confidential Enquiry into Peri-operative Deaths' has shown differences in outcome relate to the frequency a team carries out a particular operation [1]. Repetition can improve quality. Rather than trying to tackle the unfamiliar, consideration should be given to employing an expert in the field; this may mean referral to another unit. Such action can increase the patient's confidence in those making the referral.

The manager may need to consider how to increase the flexibility of staff in those fields where excellence is to be the quality target. As knowledge and medicine progress rapidly, it is more cost-effective to invest in staff education rather than training. A flexible response comes from the ability to transfer knowledge between different situations. Training is focused and, while it may provide an individual who can perform a specific job excellently, further change may leave them unable to adapt.

The directorate need to discuss which areas of their work might be improved rapidly and which could be better performed by other teams. All the team members should be consulted. The proposed changes can then be built into the outline strategy for the following year's budget. Major changes in contracts need a carefully planned lead time. Purchasers may wish to finance a higher quality of service locally rather than have to seek a service elsewhere.

The directorate needs to take a pride in offering excellence in specific areas of practice and in offering a reasonable standard in all the others.

The directorate also needs to seek new areas for development and to encourage creativity. According to Cleese (1991), creativity requires: space; time to think and refine; confidence; and some humour.

To stamp out creativity: allow no humour; undermine confidence; demand people should always be actively doing things; 'demand urgency at all times, use lots of fighting talk, establish a permanent atmosphere of stress and crisis' [2]. Managers would do well to review whether the climate they create encourages creativity.

References

1. Buck, N., Devlin, H.B. and Lunn, J. (eds) (1987) *The Report of a Confidential Enquiry into Peri-operative Deaths*, Nuffield Provincial Hospital Trust, London.
2. Cleese, J. (1991) (quoted by Anne Ferguson) *Independent on Sunday*, February 3, 1991.

Further reading

Campling, E.A., Devlin, H.B. and Lunn, J.E. (eds) (1990) *A Report of the National Confidential Enquiry into Peri-operative Deaths*, NECEPOD, 35–43 Lincoln's Inn Fields, London WC2A 3PN.
Peters, T. and Austin, N. (1985) *A Passion for Excellence: The Leadership Difference*, Fontana/Collins, England.
Peters, T. and Waterman, R.H. (1982) *In Search of Excellence*, Harper & Row, New York.

EXCUSES

Do not make them – give honest reasons.

An apology should be made, with the reason for late delivery of a report or for a mistake. Consider if some means of redress is required. No manager should insult the patient or customer, when they show concern for poor service, by dismissing their feelings and implying theirs are less important than those of the staff.

When things go wrong, as they inevitably will, observe how the staff handle the situation. Does it sound and feel like a real apology? Is the hidden message to the patient that they should be grateful for any service, however poor?

Improving the quality of how the team deal with mistakes and delays can start with including it as a topic at monthly quality meetings. It may also be useful to discuss how the hospital copes with mistakes affecting staff, for example the reaction of the pay office when it makes an error with the salaries.

F

FAIRNESS

Everyone likes to be judged on performance, not looks, personality, manners, who they know or where they trained. Discourage sexist, racist and ageist language.

Job-application forms should be checked to see if they request marital status, information about children or dependants, country of birth, religion, name of school, political affiliation, a photograph or medical history. If they do, the personnel department should be asked to revise the form to comply with a fair, equal-opportunities policy. Personal details such as marital status can be obtained from the successful applicant on the first day in post.

As a check on fairness in employment, it is helpful to ask the personnel department to produce an annual statistical review of the proportion of applicants from each racial group appointed. Managers may also consider whether job advertisements are placed in the papers read by the local ethnic minorities.

Racism is covert in the NHS. Managers must redress the balance by providing opportunities for disadvantaged staff to attend professional and management courses. Review the ways these are advertised and structured as part-time staff may be disadvantaged [2].

The uniform policy should also be examined to see if it disadvantages those from ethnic minority groups. Trousers and tunics for women may help recruitment.

Access courses may be run in partnership with local colleges of education to help those recently arrived in this country to improve their grasp of English and to gain the necessary qualifications to enter professional training.

Opportunities could be provided for work experience within the directorate.

It is vital that the wards of the directorate provide a fair deal for patients from different ethnic backgrounds. Patient-teaching aids such as videos, cassettes and leaflets in minority languages can be developed. The quality team should review whether different clothing and bathing requirements are catered for. The manager may wish to consider whether the ward and staff menus cater for all dietary requirements, such as dishes without animal products (including certain fats), kosher and halal meat. The team may wish to check whether the nursing and medical staff are aware of the characteristics and practices of the major world religions. The representative from the appropriate ethnic community should be asked to help. The Community Health Council may be able to suggest contacts with a special interest in health care. They will also have access to simple leaflets about health care in a range of languages.

The directorate may wish to consider requesting funds to employ a liaison worker to help with interpretation and health education. A list of staff or contacts who speak a foreign language and who would be willing to translate for patients or relatives should be readily available in all clinical areas. The use of a telephone language line may provide a useful resource. The quality team may also wish to look at signposting along the path that the patient would follow from the admission office to the wards. Signs with pictograms that indicate the way can be helpful to those who cannot read.

It may be helpful to plan a study programme for the staff on issues of race and culture.

Reference

1. Equal Opportunities Commission (1991) *Equality Management: Women's Employment in the NHS,* Equal Opportunities Commission, Manchester.
2. NHS Management Executive. *Ethnic Minority Staff in the NHS: A Programme of Action,* EL(94)12, Department of Health, Leeds.

Useful contact for publications and help

Commission for Racial Equality, Elliot House, 10–12 Allington Street, London SW1E 5EH.

FEEDBACK

Staff should be told the important messages and what is being planned. The manager must answer questions, listen to their ideas and 'feed it back' up the line.

A daily information meeting can be implemented and, if there are a lot of staff, it should be arranged for the information to cascade down to everyone on duty within the space of 24 hours. Some hospitals have adopted formal team briefing schemes such as that from the Industrial Society [1].

The manager may consider circulating the agreed minutes of most meetings attended. Where most of the meeting does not refer to the directorate or unit, it may be more helpful to photocopy and circulate extracts of particular interest. New appointments should be announced on noticeboards and include a little of the person's background so people will have a starting point when they later welcome the newcomer.

Feedback on individual performance is important. Consider a one minute praising [2]. Nursing and medicine in particular have long maintained control by making staff feel uncomfortable about a poor performance, rather than positively reinforcing good practice. The wise manager remembers the feeling of 'what have I done now' when summoned to the office to see a senior manager. A regular review of personal management style from time to time, particularly on the amount of coaching, can prove helpful.

References

1. Industrial Society, *Communications Skills Guide*, Industrial Society, Birmingham.
2. Blanchard, K. and Johnson, S. (1989) *The One Minute Manager*, Fontana/Collins, Glasgow.

FIRING PEOPLE

An unpleasant management task that has to be performed if the team is carrying an incompetent or disruptive member. Removing the bad performer will lift the morale of the team and improve the overall quality and reliability.

Poor performance must be dealt with whenever it occurs. Honest and timely feedback should be given. A manager should avoid the 'hit and run' style. Any local disciplinary procedure must be followed and what is said and done documented. If a teaching and coaching programme is to be undertaken it should be documented, with a copy given to the individual involved.

Dates, times, topics and objectives with a review date should be recorded. A review on the set date must take place. If the performance has not improved, the hospital policy should be used as a guide to issue the appropriate warning that dismissal is under consideration. Follow to-the-letter the detail about which officer has the authority to issue such warnings, suspend or dismiss.

Poor health, alcohol or drug dependence may affect performance. For example, poor time-keeping and failure to respond to written warnings by a domestic occurred when the GP prescribed a benzodiazepine for marital problems. Referral to the occupational health department may allow rehabilitation of a previously satisfactory worker.

The manager must be fair in assessment of performance. If in doubt about a serious incident the manager should suspend the staff involved to give time for careful investigation. Provide a clear statement of the complaint and give adequate time, both for discussion with the relevant staff representative and to prepare any defence. Provide a copy of the hospital rules and procedure for the disciplinary interview.

If a manager is concerned about conducting a disciplinary interview, a member of the personnel department whose knowledge and skills are respected can be asked to run through the procedure and areas to be explored during the interview. An analogy might be: it is like driving a car and needing to watch the road, not concentrate on the gear changes. The manager needs to be able to concentrate on the facts not the procedure.

At the end of the interview, the manager, the senior manager and the person dismissed all need to feel that every step was carried out fairly. Appeal mechanisms can take up much energy and time and a deserved dismissal can be lost on a technicality that meant the person was not treated fairly.

No person should be fired for a genuine mistake. Instead the manager should investigate exactly what went wrong and seek ways of ensuring it cannot happen again.

Quality in practice

The incorrect dose rate of an analgesic given by a syringe pump was made possible by poor design of the control screw. Investigation revealed a general lack of confidence in making up the correct drug solutions and calculating the dosage rate. Everyone learnt from the incident. The staff involved were not made the scapegoats of poor management, which can happen elsewhere.

Further reading

Croner's Employment Law Staff Editorial Department (1985) *Croner's Guide to Fair Dismissal*, 2nd edn., Croner Publications, New Malden, England.

FOCUS

On the long haul to introduce a major change in the way care is organized, alter the focus every few weeks. It stimulates staff, allows a break from concentration on one theme and may provide new insights into the previous stage of the change.

Quality in practice

When introducing the nursing process, the care plans were the despair of the ward sister. Moving to start work on the recording of the patient's response to the care and its evaluations soon led to improvements in the clarity of the wording on the plans.

FREELANCE CONSULTANTS

If staff have identified a need that only an outside consultant can meet, the manager may look around for a suitable freelance, listening to recommendations, perhaps asking advice from the professional organization or university. Some consultants send out a prospectus. It should be read with care. It is unwise to employ a consultant just because they are well-known or have had something published; writing is a different skill from helping others develop their knowledge of quality care and services. Careful thought should be given before employing someone who has worked in the hospital in a senior role, as they may be tempted to revert to it. However, they may have special expertise and knowledge of the organization that is valuable. The chosen consultant must have credibility to do the job required.

The project/study sessions should be costed carefully, including hidden costs such as staff time, the volume of paper required to carry out a survey and, if necessary, computer time. For study sessions, it helps comparability if the cost per participant is also calculated.

A detailed brief, including the objectives to be achieved, should be prepared. This can be sent out to potential consultants. If the requirements or the objectives are unclear, the manager should request a meeting with the consultant. Some may attend without charge to encourage purchase of this or future work.

Once the requirements are understood, the manager should expect a detailed proposal and a tender. This should be accompanied by a short professional profile or *curriculum vitae* to enable the manager to review the experience and knowledge being offered.

Compare the fee with the directorate's estimate. Consider the potential value to the directorate. If it is not possible to pay the asking fee the consultant should be told; it may be possible to trim the project or find cheaper ways of meeting the core requirements. Expenses may be itemized separately. If the freelance has to travel some distance, first-class rail travel may be requested to enable work to be performed during the journey.

If the freelance is to organize and present study sessions, expect the reference material and handouts to be provided as part of the charge. The manager has responsibility for providing an appropriate learning environment and in preparing the ground in order that the staff gain the maximum benefit. This includes providing aims and objectives for the session. The freelance should be given the choice of being introduced to the students or of introducing themselves. The staff should also expect to evaluate the session(s). The results can then be fed back to the freelance and the directorate can consider whether it received good value for money.

If the freelance consultant is to assist with a project to be carried out in the directorate, all the staff likely to be affected should be informed of the arrangements. The manager should also give then the opportunity to discuss any fears or concerns. The consultant or the manager should devise the project protocol. If it is to last longer than 3 months the production of an interim report should be included. The payment of fees may be staged and depend on the delivery of each report in a satisfactory format.

Writing to express appreciation of satisfactory work is helpful to the consultant. Evidence of satisfied customers can be shown to potential clients. If the work was unsatisfactory there are two options: to say nothing and not employ that person again; or to write a factual, constructive letter about the deficiencies. Care must be taken to avoid libel. Most freelance consultants wish to give of their best. If the work was less than satisfactory they may be prepared to refund part of the fee.

G

GOING GREEN

The quality of the environment is linked to every human activity. Many of those activities pollute and are harmful to health.

Review the use of aerosols – are there other equally effective preparations that do not use a propellant? When purchasing disposable items of equipment, consider the methods that will be used to dispose of them. Will the materials release toxic fumes in the incinerator or lie inert at a land-fill site? It may be necessary to request information from the manufacturer.

Review the present methods of infection control and products used for general cleaning. Inappropriate use of disinfectants may be adding permanent chemical pollutants to the waste water and can kill wildlife.

Check the procedures for the disposal of waste comply with the Health and Safety Commission guidelines. Pedal bins should have working pedals and the bags should fit into the holders. A replacement programme may be required.

Staff can be encouraged to use bicycles to get to work if there is secure storage. Patients may also need similar facilities outside the outpatients department. Changing facilities and showers should be available to staff.

The works staff could be asked to carry out an energy audit. Every room should have a wall thermometer and thermostats fitted to radiators. Areas not used every day of the week should be controlled individually. Long-life, low-energy light bulbs can be a good investment. Place stickers by each switch, with a reminder to switch off when the room is not in use. Use time-switches on cupboard lights.

Nevertheless, beware the rigid enthusiast who switches off the heating on Friday night and only switches it back on Monday, leaving the morning's patients to shiver while the rooms reheat.

Ask the supplies department to purchase recycled paper. Paper can be shredded for security and then sold for recycling. Cardboard boxes can be flattened and sent for compaction and sale. Try a collection box for patient's newspapers, cardboard chocolate boxes and used menu cards in each ward. Arrange for regular collections to limit the fire risk. Photocopy on both sides of the paper.

Glass fruit-squash bottles can be sent to the bottle banks to be recycled. Aluminium cans earn a few pence for ward funds; invest in a magnet for easy sorting from steel cans. Ask about the collection of plastics by the local authority.

Plough any income from recycling projects into trees, window boxes or tubs to brighten up the hospital grounds and improve the quality of the view for patients and staff. Buy a bird table, or a nut-holder to stick to the day-room window, to feed small birds with waste crumbs. Bird-watching with identification charts can help avoid boredom among patients.

Further reading

Alderman, C. (1990) Waging war on waste. *Nursing Standard*, **4**, 46, 22–23.

Gray, M. and Keeble, B. (1989) Greening the NHS. *British Journal of Medicine*, 299, 4–5.

Health and Safety Commission, Health Services Advisory Committee (1982) *The Safe Disposal of Clinical Waste in 1981*, HMSO, London.

NHS Management Executive (1991) *Strategic Guide to Waste Management with EL(91) M/1*, Department of Health, London.

H

HONEYMOON PERIOD

All new ideas have a honeymoon period so enjoy it! The problems will start to appear about 6 weeks after the implementation. Only presidents and prime ministers get 100 days' grace.

Introducing change raises all kinds of expectations. The manager can lead the change or act as a coach to others. All those involved need to recognize the need for the change. It helps to describe the present situation, to use the 'Man from Mars' view when thinking about 'what we think we do and what we really do', to reflect on the unintended messages that detract from the quality of technical care. Also, poor practice needs to be recognized before it can be changed. One change theory describes the need to unfreeze an activity so it can be remoulded and then frozen into the new shape.

Plan the changes with a timetable for each step. Plan for the honeymoon too. Invite potential supporters to help with the process, to find solutions to specific problems, to help find extra resources and to give emotional support during the change.

Those involved need information about the change, so consider how to provide:

- a file of relevant articles for and against the new idea;
- research reports;
- videos or films;
- a visit from a freelance 'expert';
- role play of the change.

A major change may benefit from visits to other units where the new activity is already established, to talk about the implications of the change or to work alongside the staff to get the feel for what lies ahead. Inform those outside the team through newsletters, information sheets, discussions and planning sessions.

Make the change public.

Introduce the change. Give the new ideas at least 3 months' trial. Review progress each month with the team. Help the members recognize that the excitement only lasts for a few weeks and that it can be followed by depression and dissatisfaction at the slow pace, the problems and the unfulfilled hopes. Assure them that the end of the honeymoon period in a change is anticipated and normal.

The manager should insist the trial continues, with any agreed minor modifications. These should be recorded together with the date they were introduced. The record can then be used at the end of the trial period for a careful evaluation of the benefit arising from the change. Helpful changes may become part of the routine without effort. Others may need further modification to become well-established or refrozen into the new routine.

Further reading

Spurgeon, P. and Barwell, F. (1991) *Implementing Change in the NHS,* Chapman & Hall, London.

HUMOUR

Laughter is good medicine. It releases tension and helps in facing fears.

The quality team may wish to consider having a changing display of cartoons on a noticeboard where patients pass by. The display can even become part of the therapy, as a target for the daily walking practice. Seek good quality for the jokes as in everything else.

Staff may like to compile a book of the amusing ward happenings and sayings. Many an accident-and-emergency department has a list of the odd self-diagnoses proffered by patients. However, it is important that the manager encourages staff to laugh with patients, not at them.

The team may wish to use humour to liven up notices requesting safe practice. Use the international symbols and alongside add a second copy with a local interpretation.

Change the wording or the second picture at intervals to maintain interest.

Other sites for humour and cartoons include menus, information sheets, patient education booklets and files of ward information.

The manager should seek out hidden talent. We found a management accountant who was always sketching on the blotter during lengthy meetings. The cartooned posters we commissioned from him, for the College of Nursing, greatly increased the attendance at the Open Day.

Further reading

Carlisle, D. (1990) Comic relief. *Nursing Times,* **86,** 38, 50–51.

I

INTEGRITY

Personal integrity is tied up with a person's value system. It is about the way a person behaves in daily life – practising what is preached. Honesty, consistency, wholeness – it is something special.

Many of the items outlined in this book reflect on a manager's integrity, such as **staff appraisal**, **counselling**, and **firing people**. They should be carried out honestly and without prejudice. An effective manager has empathy for others, keeps his or her own counsel, does not gossip, 'curry favour' or seek popularity for its own sake. Acting in this way the manager maintains personal integrity and does not damage others unfairly or thoughtlessly.

Integrity for the health service requires effort to deliver an honest, consistent, unified service, with each of the components neatly dovetailed into others. It should be a seamless service that provides for the entire episode of the patient's illness. Such a service is seen as high quality and usually requires the efforts of several teams, or the expansion of a team to provide care in every setting through which the patient may pass.

INVENTORY

The manager takes responsibility for the management of resources. The management of ward stocks are delegated to the ward teams, particularly where the budget has been devolved to ward level. A formal inventory of high-cost items is a requirement as they represent part of the business assets of the hospital [1]. Nevertheless, one for the smaller items of ward equipment is also helpful. Store cupboards should be kept secure, as pilfering is a constant risk in a building open to the public. New items of equipment should be marked with the ward name; invisible marking with the hospital post-code may be helpful in tracing those high-cost items more likely to be stolen.

The time-honoured method of recording items borrowed or loaned by wards is a small record book noting the date, item taken and by whom (see **Control – equipment**).

In the month following stock-taking, staff may be more conscientious in their recording; however, this tends to tail off. The wily manager may wish to stimulate awareness by carrying out spot checks.

To complete an inventory requires stock-taking. All clinical equipment and furniture should be counted, along with soft furnishings. An annual inventory of linen, blankets and pillows may be undertaken by laundry staff. Borrowed equipment should be returned and loaned items collected. Recent purchases should be added to the list and any missing items identified. The hospital-asset register requires a description of the item, its location, year of acquisition and cost, repair dates and cost of the repair.

The stock-taking exercise is also a good time to check the condition of the stock, and to plan to replace or repair items. The annual budget may have to include an allocation to enable this plan to be carried out. The location and facilities for the storage of equipment should also be reviewed. Reorganizing locations may save staff time and effort and sometimes speed up the delivery of emergency care. An annual stock-take may be combined with the annual safety check.

There are two ways of approaching the inventory: manual recording or using a hand-held or lap-top computer. Both forms of recording should be performed when activity levels are low, such as at a weekend. The route around a ward should be systematic. Manual recording may be against a handwritten or typed register or a list generated from a central computer record. The hand-held computer can hold the list of stock and be updated during the tour of the rooms. Some areas are introducing adhesive barcodes to label items and these can be read by a 'pen' with the data transferred straight into the computer.

Stocks of disposable equipment, medical and surgical supplies can also be bar-coded to enable rapid stock-taking and re-ordering. Where ordering has to be peformed manually it may be helpful to establish a set level of stock so that the task can be delegated to the ward clerk or another member of staff to top-up to the set level. A review of the levels of stock and the range held should include checking that items: are used in date rotation; are still within the expiry date; are stored in such a way that the risk of damage to protective packaging is reduced; and are still required [2].

References

1. Department of Health (1989) *Capital Charges*. Working paper 5, Working for Patients Series, HMSO, London.
2. Denton, I. (1991) Taking stock. *Nursing Times*, **87**, 46, 32–33.

J

JOB DESCRIPTIONS

A job description lists the role and responsibilities of the job in general terms. A role specification is less detailed.

Changes in the organization of clinical work, support services and the management of the directorate should be reflected in the job descriptions. They also provide both employee and manager with a starting point for the individual performance review.

When preparing a job description, the manager should look at the areas of the job that carry particular responsibilities for the quality of patient care, such as communication with others and the development of personal skills and those of other staff. Use those as the main objectives for the post and then list the key tasks for achieving them. Another approach is to write the standard of performance as one column on one side of the page and the required actions alongside in a second column.

Keep it short. Too-detailed a job description inhibits creativity and enthusiasm. Seek advice from the personnel department on the grading comparability of unusual posts, particularly those for administrative or clerical staff.

Review it with the occupant during each performance review. Remember that the clinical grading system for nurses fixes the grade to the job. Good people should consistently achieve the optimum quality of performance and grow out of the job as their knowledge and skills develop. Encourage them to seek promotion or further training.

No one should be tempted to massage the job description to fit the next grade. It is not fair, it will change the balance of the team and create resentment in other staff.

If the job genuinely has to change beyond recognition, revise the job description when the change occurs. Review the job descriptions of all the other team members. Assess the knock-on effects. If the new job is still needed, submit them all for grading.

Further reading

Ungerson, B. (1983) *How to Write a Job Description,* Institute of Personnel Management, London.

JOBSHARE

Sharing a leadership role, such as a ward-sister/charge-nurse post, requires people who can complement each other's skills, interests and knowledge. A sense of humour and mutual liking and respect are desirable. The job sharers should first agree the broad strategy. Decisions have to be made on the spot and consultation in advance is tedious. Those key tasks of the post that do not need daily attention may be divided between the two incumbents.

A manager should avoid dividing staff loyalties by favouring one of the pair. A weekly overlap should be provided so that planning and feedback can be shared with the manager.

The most appropriate posts for jobshares are those where: the period of patient contact is limited, such as day surgery, investigation units, labour wards and theatres; or so intense it needs to be limited to allow time for staff to recover as in intensive care settings.

The directorate may wish to create jobshares to provide opportunities for experienced staff to combine part-time work with study or child care.

Further reading

Buchan, J. (1991) Job share, a share in the future. *Nursing Times,* **87**, 23, 32–33.

Editorial (1987) Flexible friends. *Nursing Standard,* **2**, 30.

Hartley, S. and James, H. (1989) Child's play (job share a night-sister post). *Nursing Standard,* **3**, 36–37.

Meager, N. and Buchan, J. (1989) *Job sharing in the NHS. Report No. 174,* Institute of Manpower Studies, Brighton.

K

KEEPING IN TOUCH

Plan to spend one morning or afternoon each week working in a clinical area in order to talk with the clients but mainly to listen. The modern manager examines the system from the inside in order to identify the irritations of the organization and how they affect the patients and staff. A regular spell on night duty will complete the picture where a 24-hour service is offered.

The manager with a real interest in quality uses the hospital dining facilities provided for staff and patients:

- observe whether the service fits in with the dips in ward workload or whether it forces staff to take their break at an inconvenient time;
- notice whether relatives are allowed to use the same dining areas and whether they are made welcome – this may be particularly important for parents resident on site in order to be close to a sick child;
- consider whether the special needs of night staff are recognized and met;
- check the range of foods available to see that healthy eating is possible by night and day.

When staff leave for a career break or further professional training, the manager should consider keeping in contact and helping them to keep in touch with developments in the directorate and hospital. It may be possible to join with other managers to compile a regular newsletter to send out to them, or to send on a copy of the hospital news sheet with the directorate's minutes of meetings.

Invitations to study sessions, ward outings and parties help reinforce old ties. Staff on career breaks may feel much happier about coming back to work part-time or on the hospital 'bank' if they remain familiar with the jargon and hear about the changes first-hand. The manager should consider lending out videos of clinical topics, self-directed learning packages and any educational packages developed by the team.

Adjust the budget to allow a scheme for those on a longer career break to return on a planned basis to work for 1–2 weeks each year to update their hands-on skills. A short structured programme will allow the maximum value to be extracted from the experience. A temporary place in a local crèche or nursery that coincides with the holiday of another member of the team who uses the facility can ease childcare problems. Another option is to plan the dates so that older children can attend the hospital school-holiday play scheme.

Further reading

Fitzgerald, M. (1989) Will ye no come back? *Nursing Times*, **85**, 24, 54–55.

L

LEADERSHIP

While the quality of the performance is the personal responsibility of each member of the team, there is a role for the leader to point out the direction and set the pace. Not all people in leadership positions will lead. Leaders make efforts to shape change, while their weaker colleagues just accommodate the changes imposed by others, are reactive and less imaginative.

According to Tom Peters and Nancy Austin:

> Leadership means vision, cheerleading, enthusiasm, love, trust, verve, passion, obsession, consistency, the use of symbols, paying attention as illustrated by the content of one's calendar, out and out drama (and the management thereof), creating heroes at all levels, coaching, effectively wandering around, and numerous other things. [1]

A well-led team consistently achieves quality in performance. When the best leader's work is done the people say 'We did it ourselves.'

Leaders are needed at all levels. Clinical practice, research and education need effective leaders as well as in management. The effective manager invests time and resources in developing potential among the staff, developing a reputation for talent-spotting and channelling the energies of the rebels. It attracts further good people to spend time working in the directorate and enhances its reputation.

Reference

1. Peters, T. and Austin, N. (1985) *A Passion for Excellence*, Fontana/Collins, Glasgow.

Further reading

Bennis, W. and Nanus, B. (1985) *Leaders: The Strategies for Taking Charge*, Harper & Row, New York.

Christman, L. (1987) A view to the future. *Nursing Outlook*, **35**, 5, 216–18.

LEADERSHIP STYLES

There are two main styles of leadership behaviour – directing and supporting. When directing, the manager clearly sets out the 'what', 'how', 'where' and 'when' of the task and supervises its performance. Supporting behaviour requires listening, encouraging ideas and involving staff in problem-solving and decisions.

Blanchard *et al.* [1] gives four leadership styles:

- **Directing** – high direction, low support;
- **Coaching** – high direction, high support;
- **Supporting** – low direction, high support;
- **Delegating** – low direction, low support.

In hospitals, the manager may use the directing style when the person lacks competence but is enthusiastic and committed. Performance expectations have to be simple, clear, consistent and concrete. The student or new member of the team will benefit from this style to get started. Some people, who because of their experience of life have lost confidence in themselves, may seek the security of being directed. Institutionalization can do this to patients and staff. Dips in the overall quality scores in a ward can coincide with a major changeover of staff. The wise manager anticipates the temporary need for greater direction and allocates staff, who can use the directing style, to teach the newcomers.

Values are shaped by direction when new to the job. A tough task master who values excellence yet gives due praise will influence quality. This is face-to-face leadership for high quality.

Coaching styles are useful when there is developing competence but a lack of commitment, or to build experience and self esteem. It is helpful when the 'honeymoon period' of a key change has come to an end. Consistent standards are required. The manager's actions must fit the words.

A supporting style helps when there is competence but lack of confidence or motivation. The manager has to listen, praise and facilitate. The limits set to stretch performance must be achievable. Staff returning after a career break or a tour abroad need this style of leadership for a few weeks.

Delegating is most appropriate when the staff have competence and commitment. The low support, low-direction content are still needed, or the person will feel abandoned with the manager abdicating responsibility.

A manager needs to develop flexibility in order to move between the four leadership styles as the person's competence develops in a role or at a task. New tasks may require direction while familiar ones might be delegated. The annual performance review should include an exchange of opinion over which style the manager should use for each of the four or five objectives.

The manager should also review the leadership styles of the staff. They can be changed through counselling, education and training. The overall styles of ward sisters received attention in the 1980s. Fleishman's leadership opinion questionnaire was used to assess the styles of managers in a range of occupations. This has two independent scores: structure and consideration.

Consideration scores reflect the extent to which a manager is likely to have job relationships with subordinates characterized by mutual trust, respect for their ideas, consideration for their feelings and a certain warmth. A high score indicates good rapport and two-way communications. A low score indicates a more impersonal approach.

Structure scores reflect the extent to which the individual is likely to define their role and that of subordinates towards goal attainment. The activities include planning, communicating information, scheduling, criticizing and trying out new ideas.

It was found [2] that high structure scores were needed when there was uncertainty or the introduction of change such as the nursing process, or a move to new operating theatres.

The ideal surgical ward sister also needed high scores to give students a feeling of security in the uncertain period of post-operative recovery.

High consideration scores were found among medical ward sisters, particularly where the staff were experienced in that type of nursing, or the pace of change in the patient's condition was slow.

In the eyes of the student nurses, the ideal ward sister had a high consideration score and a moderate structure score. The sisters most successful in implementing the nursing process had high structure scores and high consideration scores. Repeat studies showed change over time, with increasing scores for consideration. Counselling and further professional education helped them flex their general styles to the ward needs. Major changes to increase the quality of care through adjusting procedures or the ward organization will require similar variations in leadership styles.

New staff also need to consider the overall style of the leader. Ogier and Barnett [3] found that the structure and consideration scores of staff nurses were closer to those of the ward sister, the longer they worked together.

References

1. Blanchard, K., Zigarmi, P. and Zigarmi, D. (1985) *Leadership and the One Minute Manager*, Fontana/Collins, Glasgow.
2. Ogier, M.E. (1982) *An Ideal Sister?* Royal College of Nursing, London.
3. Ogier, M.E. and Barnett, D.E. (1985) Sister, staff nurse, nurse learner. *Nurse Education Today*, **6**, 16–22.

Further reading

Ogier, M.E. and Barnett, D.E. (1985) Unhappy learners ahead? *Nursing Mirror*, **161**, 3, 18–20.

LISTS

Agree with the ward teams, two lists of equipment with prices that would be most useful. One list of items under £100, the other list of more expensive items. Keep these with a file of the current manufacturer's information on each one.

Use the file when there is a sudden opportunity to put in an unexpected bid or to react to the offer of a gift from a grateful patient or charity. An item can also be selected if there is a safety net of money unspent at the end of the 3-month period (see **Budgets**). It is wiser not to wait beyond 3 months as another department's overspends could see year-end cuts applied to everyone and the whole nest-egg taken away.

Prepare an information file of the important things ward staff need to know and which are not included in the policy or procedure manuals. Lists of contacts, emergency action, sources of emergency supplies and so on can be kept in a handy file or on the ward computer for easy access. On notice boards they quickly become tatty and may be covered by posters or more recent notices.

The IHSM yearbook [1] provides a source of lists of statutory instruments, circulars from the Department of Health, Scottish Office, Welsh Office and Northern Ireland, addresses of health authorities and senior officers, and health service bibliographies.

Lists can also help in solving problems. All the factors should be listed and then arranged in order of importance relative to the problem. Vilfredo Pareto, a 19th-century economist, discovered that most of the welfare was in the hands of the vital few, while the vast majority (the trivial many) existed in poverty. Pareto's principle can be applied to the problems by dividing the list into the vital few and working on them first.

The principle also works for stocks, such as dressings. Keep only the 'vital few' in the store – it is surprising how the 'trivial many' can be replaced by a creative use of those vital few.

Another way to use lists for decision-making is to list the alternative solutions, compare these for the long- and short-term gains and also the spin-offs they would offer. Then rate the risk of problems occurring with each one.

Plans to improve quality can be divided into lists of action required immediately, in the mid-term and by gradual progression, by small steps, to the long term. The list can be divided into the 'can do now' from the 'needs preparation' items. The tasks can also be broken down into small chunks.

The most important step is to start work.

Reference

1. I HSM (1993) *The Hospitals and Health Services Year Book 1993*, Institute of Health Services Management, 75 Portland Place, London W1N 4AN.

M

MAN FROM MARS

Once in a while the manager should stand back from the work and pretend to be a little green 'man/woman from Mars'.

What would he/she make of the wards and departments and the way in which they are run? What hidden messages might he/she see in the way staff and managers greet and talk with the patients and their visitors?

The man/woman from Mars technique differs from the 'fly on the wall' through its use of the alien perspective to interpret everyday activities. It is an aid to lateral thinking and innovation.

MANAGEMENT ACCOUNTANT

Every manager's main concern should be with the future – laying foundations today for the developments of tomorrow. The management accountant is concerned with the financial future, predicting the economic consequences and resource implications of the manager's decisions.

As the technical expert with mathematics, he or she should be representing activity in mathematical models. To simulate the different options – the 'what if?' predictions – to help the manager predict and therefore plan.

Activities have to be identified. The manager has to help by supplying information:

- Is the cost fixed or does it vary?
- What relationship does the activity have to the cost?
- Is there a pattern?
- Could it be used to predict future costs of quality improvements?

Every new policy carries with it a cost. It may be as simple as the reimbursement cost of a vial of hepatitis B vaccine used to protect staff at risk. Or the cost of vaccine, occupational health nurse time, syringes and needles to give the vaccine to staff at risk. A different cost again if it is to be offered to all the staff. The management accountant can do the sums, perhaps also working out the potential savings from reduced staff sickness from hepatitis B. The manager makes the decision. The management accountant provides the information on the cost of each option in more than financial terms.

Cost accounting can look back at an activity and work out what it really cost. Cost centres are used to track down who spent the money. The aim is for each ward to become a cost centre for specific resources. Analysis of variance can help the manager track down reasons for changes in actual expenditure compared with the plans.

Treasure the management accountant. Most have a strong interest in patient care and can help the clinical manager to get enhanced value from the allocated budget.

Quality in practice

The budget for incontinence pads went into the red. The analysis showed which month the trend began. It was not due to an increase in the number of patients with incontinence. On investigation it was shown to be the Supplies Department making a saving per pad by a change to a cheaper brand. The pads were less absorbent so more frequent changes had to be used to keep the patients dry and comfortable. There was also an increase in the nursing workload. The Management Accountant's hard facts held sway where the ward nurse's opinions had failed to convince the Supplies Manager of the problem. The new brand was cancelled.

Further reading

Harper, W.M. (1989) *Management Accounting*, Longman, London.

MANAGERS

The most effective managers work in the ward or department alongside their staff for part of every week. That way they can listen to the views of patients, observe for problems and spot areas for improvement. Management by wandering around (MBWA) has been the vogue for managers in manufacturing and commercial companies for some years. It is not the same as 'keeping your hand in' in order to be able to give practical help in a crisis.

Clinical credibility helps the manager fight for the required resources.

If the problems need a quick answer it is asking for too much effort to have to be contacted at the end of a bleep or telephone. To be there when needed is a skill. Around too much and the staff feel they are not trusted. Beware of the manager who never seems to go home. The manager who goes home at the end of the day, leaving a 'phone number in case a big problem comes up will find that it is not used very much but staff feel secure. Big problems should be very infrequent! In the same way the 'phone numbers of the team should be held by their manager in case of an emergency.

MEASURING QUALITY

Only some aspects of quality are directly measurable; these include those listed in Table 1.

Other qualities may be judged as present or absent, based on patient or professional opinion against agreed descriptions of what is desired. This can include a checklist of standards or indicators, questionnaires or surveys. These are not directly measurable qualities. All that can be indicated numerically is the proportion judged to be present. Too often the ill-informed treat such results as if they were scientific facts. They then run the risk of basing their actions on a foundation akin to unstable sand, rather than solid rock. Retesting will be equally inaccurate, so the results of their remedial action are unclear.

Information to aid measurement may be obtained from one or more of the following sources:

- Records of clinical treatment;
- Accident report forms;
- Interviews of patients and significant others;
- Observation of the patient, care and environment;
- Observation of staff performance;
- Identification of available resources;
- Budget statements.

Table 1 Aspects of quality that are measurable directly and examples

Quality attribute	Examples
Time	The time taken to carry out an activity
	Length of stay
	Length of wait after an appointment time
	Waiting time for non-urgent admission.
Frequency	Number of times an activity is carried out in 24 hours
	Unplanned-admission rates.
Regularity	Actual times a prescribed regular activity is carried out
	2-hourly changes of position
Temperature	In different environments
	Variations throughout the 24 hours
Size	Skin loss
	Decubitous ulcers
	Number of patients with a specific complication
Proportion	Percentage of patients with a specific infection from the total undergoing a particular operation
	Number with a specific complaint

Start small. Take care in **selecting tools to measure quality**. The subjects to be measured may be chosen because they are giving cause for concern, such as poor communications, or to assess an innovation, new equipment or strategy. Any tool, chosen or designed locally, should be used systematically and at set intervals. However some high-priority qualities could be selected for random periodic re-measurement or regular sampling.

Measuring quality can identify good practice with desirable outcomes and reinforce its use as a model for others.

Further reading

Alderman, C. (1990) An agenda for change. *Nursing Standard*, **4**, 41, 54–55.

Kings Fund Institute (1989) *Briefing paper No. 9: Managed Competition*, Kings Fund Institute, London.

Kitson, A. (1986) Quality assurance – the methods of measuring quality. *Nursing Times*, **August 27**, 32–34.

Sale, D. (1990) Quality assurance, in: *Essentials of Nursing Management*, Macmillan, London.

Savage, J. (1990) Promoting good practice. *Nursing Standard*, **4**, 41, 52–53.

MEASURING PERFORMANCE

Performance is the amount made or produced or done in relation to the resources used to make or produce or do it. It is output per unit of input. It is not simply output (or outcome, or activity or throughput); nor is it simply input (or resource or cost), it is the ratio of one to the other [1].

Performance indicators now known as health service indicators have been used for several years by regional and district managers to compare the performance and resources within and between districts. They are presented as ratios to compare the number of staff to patients, bed occupancy and length of stay in particular specialities, discharges and deaths, and capital costs. They can also be used as a management tool by the hospital or directorate to identify needs and as a stimulus for action. However, that action needs to be monitored to ensure that in seeking to solve one problem, another is not created, for example, spending money to improve quality for one client group may inadvertently deprive another. Before taking any action, the manager should examine the overall objectives of the directorate and the hospital and how changes may impinge on them.

The directorate should rank the needs in order of priority, develop an action plan and decide what will give the greatest benefit.

Measurable aspects include:

- **Time**:
    the time taken to intubate a patient;
    the time taken to complete a task correctly.
- **Frequency**:
    post-catheterisation urine infection;
    alterations to the operating list.

- **Regularity**:
  actual time the vital signs are recorded;
  actual times at which the prescribed medication is administered.
- **Proportion**:
  of errors in drug administration;
  of correct answers in a clinical knowledge test.
- **Skills**:
  blood pressure level from external cardiac massage on a 'Resusci Annie' doll.

Interviews and questionnaires for patients' and carers' opinions of the care received and suggestions for improvement may indicate excellent or poor performance by one or more members of the team. The Department of Health has issued guidance on the conduct of consumer surveys in a series of booklets produced by the Centre for Health Economics at York University [2].

Individual Performance Review (IPR) is now the method commonly used to assess performance against criteria or objectives agreed between the individual member of staff and the manager. This review takes place on a regular basis, usually once a year.

Managers should make sure they understand the purpose and procedure for the review; they should familiarize themselves with the guidelines and the forms. They should also ensure all involved staff have attended study sessions on the system. If there are no suitable guidelines to help staff prepare for the review, the manager should compile a set for the directorate.

Both manager and the interviewee should know what is expected of them. An appointment should be made well in advance; this will give both parties time to think about the performance. The interviewee should also consider what is desired from the organization and the manager in particular. The chosen venue for the meeting should be free of interruptions and enough time given to the review for it to be useful: up to 3 hours may need to be set aside.

The manager needs to consider the quality of the review process. If it has been successful, the member of staff being interviewed should leave the meeting feeling positive about work, knowing what is required in the coming months, what help will be provided and any time limits for action.

Apart from the assessment carried out by professional bodies to award certificates, diplomas and degrees, there are not many systems available to measure individual clinical performance.

Peer review is a process whereby people of equal qualification and grade subjectively assess the performance of one of their peers. It may be carried out by a specific committee or a group of staff from a particular ward. The purpose may be to:

- give an assessment of the performance of an individual, guided by standards and criteria;
- identify areas for improvement;
- assess suitability for promotion or merit awards.

Peer review can be influential in changing attitudes and behaviour. However, to be effective the terms should be clear and the process seen as fair. It is not something to be undertaken lightly. A protocol must be developed, the procedure laid down, standards set and the method for dealing with the results agreed. As with all innovations, consultation and effective communications are necessary and the rules covering confidentiality respected. The innovation must be piloted before final acceptance of the protocol.

Medical audit findings may have repercussions for other disciplines so the manager should be aware of the procedure used for dealing with the findings. Clinical audit allows more direct involvement of all the health care staff and is therefore the preferred method once each discipline is confident in using the audit procedures.

Quality monitoring tools tend to focus on the process of care delivery rather than the outcome. Process standards indicate the level of staff performance expected by patients, colleagues and the employer. Standards are a means of demonstrating the values and skills of the individual and of the team. In devising descriptions of the desired performance the starting point is a clarification of what the practitioner actually does. The focus of measuring performance may include:

- observing or timing care as it is given, and the preparation for clinical procedures;
- asking questions of the staff, patients and family/carers;
- checking clinical records and available resources.

The relevant professional organizations or trade unions may provide additional advice on good practice. The wise manager informs them at an early stage in the development of standards and keeps them informed of progress.

References

1. Harper, J. (1986) Measuring performance – a new approach. *Hospital and Health Services Review*, **9**, **January**, 26–28.
2. Donn, M. (1990) Listen and learn. *Health Service Journal*, **100**, **May 10**, 701.

Further reading

Black, N., Chapple, D., Dalziel, M. and Spilby, J. (1989) Step by step to audit. *Health Service Journal*, **February 2**, 140–41.
Buchan, J. (1990) Paying for performance. *Nursing Standard*, **4**, 21, 44–45.
Fitzgibbon, M. (1986) *Quality assurance and nursing peer review*, Smith and Nephew Florence Nightingale Scholarship Study Tour Report, The Florence Nightingale Committee, London.
Kitson, A. (1986) Quality assurance – the method of measuring quality. *Nursing Times*, **27**, 32–4.
Mullins, A.C., Colavecchio, R.E. and Tescher, B.E. (1979) Peer review: a model for professional accountability. *Journal of Nursing Administration*, **December**, 25–30.
Nelson, M.J. (1989) *Managing Health Professionals*, Chapman & Hall, London.

MEETINGS

Keep them short.

Assignments

Informal or formal meetings to assign specific work require planning to make the maximum use of the time spent. They can be used to get things achieved by, through or with others. At the end of the set time agree the date and time of the next meetings to consider progress.

Daily staff meeting for information

Same place, same time. Start on time no matter who is missing and make brief notes in the diary/communications book so that those not present are also informed.

Monthly quality review

Same time, same place each month. Agree dates for the coming year so that duty rotas can be adjusted. Have a set time to finish that is adhered to. A meeting open to anyone in the directorate who can get there. An agenda, prepared so that nothing is forgotten, and read out at the start of the meeting.

Before the quality meeting, the manager should arrange for one person to make brief notes on each area of quality to be addressed, together with the name of the volunteer who agreed to lead the action. The action column on formal minutes can be used to record the name against the item.

For each of the most recent reports on quality or published reports relevant to the work of the directorate, the manager should ask one person to prepare a 2-minute verbal summary, which sets out the key points. The whole group can then spend 5 minutes brainstorming ideas on what changes are needed within the directorate. A flip-chart can be used to record the ideas. Two volunteers can work on these ideas and come up with recommendations. These can be discussed with the manager a week later. The volunteers then take responsibility for sounding out their colleagues' views on the proposals and later for over-seeing the implementation.

If a topic creates much fervour during a meeting, the manager should sum up the views expressed and move on to the next item. Those who will differ in public are unlikely to accept defeat in public. It is therefore unhelpful to dwell on a difference of opinion in a meeting. The change should be negotiated in private.

At monthly meetings the focus should be on progress and only refer to difficulties with ideas that are still being implemented if these have not been covered in the daily information meetings.

A review of whether the meeting continues to be necessary should be carried out at least once a year, or when attendance declines. The review should cover what has been achieved, work still incomplete or waiting to be started. If the meetings are not achieving action, they should be stopped and the time spent on meetings used to achieve the desired outcome in a different way.

Further reading

Gordon, M. (1985) *How to Plan and Conduct a Successful Meeting*, Sterling Publishing Co., New York.

MISTAKES

Everyone makes them. Learn from them. Good judgement is the product of experience, experience is the product of bad judgement. Too often an organization seeks to recruit experienced staff, yet at the same time tries to create settings bound up with procedure books, detailed policies and rules.

The sin in quality management should be in playing safe, not in innovation. Many surgical operations have come from taking risks, learning from mistakes, and all with the co-operation of patients who felt that when life was threatened, any risk was better than sure death. If the gamble did not pay off, at least what had been learnt would reduce the risk for the next person.

The manager should be humble and admit mistakes, identify the lesson learned and expect of staff that they do the same. A manager who talks about personal mistakes can give the staff the message that errors from trying to improve are acceptable.

MONITORING

Monitoring is an activity carried out by every manager or by someone to whom management has delegated specific authority to observe, adjust a process, instruct staff or admonish them if their work falls outside agreed limits.

It uses the formal management structure for quality control. It is different from self-control; it is carried out by staff empowered to make changes based on the results of quality management and audit.

Informal monitoring can be performed when walking around wards. It can be listening to the hospital 'grapevine' for coded messages that there are problems, for example with the performance of particular staff.

Formal monitoring may be performed by:

- the manager;
- the staff from the quality assurance department;
- selected senior members of the ward team.

It can be carried out by listing the activities to be monitored, organizing a rota of specific subjects, for example, monthly questionnaires to the ward sister/charge nurse about the level of satisfaction with the domestic service or comments from patient questionnaires. To be effective, the monitors need a comprehensive education and training programme (see **Educating – quality**).

The person monitoring quality may work alone, with another, or as part of an audit group. Selecting the right people to do the monitoring is crucial: 'they should have a commitment to quality, clinical credibility, the ability to make objective judgements and to report accurately on what they observe' [1]. They should have sufficient professional sensitivity to abandon the monitoring visit if the ward situation so demands it, for example if there was an extreme shortage of staff.

Staff should be kept informed about the implementation of formal quality assurance systems. Ensure that they have access to the quality monitoring materials that will be used. This enables the staff to understand the purpose and procedure of monitoring and subsequent findings.

Use a list of standards and/or criteria, objectives, or indicators to guide observation and thus judgements. The observations can require a response that is scored to produce a numerical result. Care must be taken to avoid such results being mistaken for factual measurements.

The information that the monitor checks or assesses can be obtained from one or a combination of the following sources:

- patient and nurse records;
- patient or carer interview;
- staff interview;
- observation of the patient, his/her care and environment;
- observation of practice and its management;
- the provision of support services.

The frequency of monitoring activities depends on the needs of the directorate and hospital. It is influenced by what is to be monitored and why.

Formal monitoring should be regular and on an agreed date. If using a checklist or quality monitoring tool, consideration should be given to using it every 4 months to allow sufficient time to correlate findings and to give the ward staff time to implement an action plan to improve quality.

Quality monitoring may be an annual activity to review compliance with provider contracts, to review the effectiveness of budget planning; or monitoring the quality of patient care received by specific groups. Quarterly monitoring may cover accident reports and complaints or the use of a quality monitoring tool. Monthly monitoring may cover infection control rates; reviewing patient dependency categorization including 'throughput', length of stay and percentage of day cases.

It is important that quality scores are given to staff as soon as possible after the formal monitoring has taken place. Time should be made available to discuss the results. While there is a need to deal with the low scores, there is also a need to acknowledge the areas of high quality. Any 'not-applicable' responses should be examined; for example, where the facilities or staff were not available but should have been, the response should have been negative, so reducing the score rather than giving a falsely high score.

A monitor should record the findings, the team's response and action plan and the manager's views on resources required. This provides an *aide memoire* for monitoring the results from appraising quality.

The monitoring approach requires the manager to give instructions on the improvements required, and to ensure through management action that these are carried out.

Practical points

One evening a monitor was particularly impressed by a patient care plan she had randomly selected. The record was well-written, stating the patient had had a good day and was now resting. However, when the monitor went to look for the patient, she discovered that he had been discharged the previous day.

The moral of the story for the ward nurse lies in checking with the patient before writing notes and always to write the truth.

The moral for the monitor is to first check the patient is available before spending time checking the paperwork. The general moral is that quality monitoring must not depend on written records alone.

Reference

1. Kemp, N. (1986) What is quality assurance? *Professional Nurse*, **1**, 124–26.

Further reading

Kendall, H. (1990) Monitoring standards of care. *Nursing Standard*, **4**, 37, 32–33.

Sale, D. (1990) *Quality Assurance*, Essentials of Nursing Management Series, Macmillan, London.

NHS Training Directorate (1993) *Monitoring the Patients' Charter: Good Practice Guide* and *Monitoring Made Easy*, NHS Training Directorate, Bristol.

MORALE

Morale is about confidence in oneself, the team and the hospital. It affects the general climate of each ward and department in a directorate.

Low morale is indicated by bickering, lack of interest in ward activities such as poor attendance at meetings and social events, refusal to co-operate in change, conspiracy and open conflict with management. The performance of individuals declines, fatigue sets in, sickness and absence rates rise and the staff turnover increases.

This has a knock-on effect on patient care; length of stay is longer as Revans [1] demonstrated so clearly. The manager should compare the rates for the directorate with similar units in other hospitals, the health service indicators providing a starting point for this.

The performance-review system can be used to identify career aspirations and to seek opportunities to develop staff within the wards. Women, in particular, may have low self-esteem, so assertiveness training should be considered. Smart uniforms should not be underestimated as morale-boosters for both sexes. They can also contribute to a corporate image.

Effective management raises morale. Clear objectives for the team, the delegation of important tasks, a willingness to listen to staff views and to tackle long-standing problems, however minor, all convey the message that the manager values the contribution of staff.

Any individual decline in performance should be discussed in an empathetic and supportive way with the individual. It may be caused by a personal problem, which will respond to counselling. Honest, constructive criticism, given in private, with clear targets for the required change in behaviour are more effective than tolerating poor quality work.

The directorate should celebrate good work and praise effort, providing staff and patients with positive 'strokes' of recognition.

Practical points

One senior manager was proud he was 'single-minded and only concerned with the business in hand'. He showed this by not acknowledging staff as he passed them in the corridors or dining room. He liked to convey that he was too busy planning what he was going to say at his next big meeting.

None of the staff went out of their way to be loyal towards him or to support his innovations. Although he dealt fairly with individuals, they thought he lacked interest in them as people and felt too superior to speak to them. Not surprisingly, team morale was low but he could not understand why!

Reference

1. Revans, R.W. (1976) *Action Learning in Hospitals*, McGraw-Hill, Maidenhead.

Further reading

Nelson, M.J. (1989) *Managing Health Professionals*, Chapman & Hall, London.
Ng, C. (1991) Work attendance study. *Senior Nurse*, **11**, 4, 12–16.
Shepperdson, B. (1990) Why nurses leave their jobs: clinical recruitment. *Nursing Times*, **4**, 22, 27–30.

MOTIVATION

Motivation is the result of internal processes. The manager should foster self-motivation, self-assessment and self-confidence among the staff by creating a work environment that challenges, invigorates and lets everyone have fun at work achieving improvements.

Our recent culture seems to imply that there is nothing between winning and losing, and that money is the only measure of success. Managers can make a stand for quality. Success is doing one's best.

Set targets and keep a score of the team's achievements.

Consider having a notice announcing results, such as how many days have elapsed since the last clean wound became infected, the last pressure sore was found in the ward.

Patients are also a part of the team working to improve their own health with the support of the staff. Care plans set individual targets for improvement. Consider celebrating patient achievements with medals, certificates and badges; give a boost to learning to walk again, moving the bowels for the first time after surgery for piles (haemorrhoids) or remembering to perform breathing exercises on time, every day, without a reminder. Small human achievements deserve at least a hug of congratulation.

The British tradition of keeping a 'stiff upper lip' in the face of adversity requires sensitivity from the staff in which method of motivation is selected for the individual patient.

Further reading

Adair, J. (1990) *Understanding Motivation*, Talbot Adair Press, Guildford.
Keating, K. (1983) *Little Book of Hugs*, Angus & Robertson, London.

N

NEGOTIATION

Negotiation is required when there are two or more parties with different views and values about a joint activity.

Patients and ward staff may negotiate a plan of care acceptable to both but not fully meeting the requirements of either. The vagrant who refuses the recommended daily bath may agree to two baths a week for the comfort of staff and other patients.

Negotiations with staff representatives may be required when changes to improve the quality of patient care will alter or affect adversely the working practices, hours or conditions of other staff groups.

Effective negotiations require preparation. Collect the facts, consider the range of options available and identify the most desirable, the acceptable and the impossible. Consider the probable response of the other side to each of these options. Draw up a list of the issues common to the desirable and acceptable options.

Staff representatives should be provided with a broad outline of the facts and the initial proposal (most desirable option). Request a preliminary meeting to clarify the proposal in order that the representative can then seek staff views and prepare for the main meetings.

The first negotiating meeting should start with the manager stating the general problem and asking the other side if they feel able to accept any of the proposal or if they have an alternative solution. If either is acceptable there is no need to negotiate. If not, at least both sides know the two starting points. Discuss each issue, one at a time.

An effective negotiator is open to the other party's views and is prepared to give a little at a time to achieve a solution acceptable to both sides. It must not be assumed that because the representative comes from a different discipline, there are no shared values about the quality of care to be offered to patients and staff. Discuss the way each proposal would help the ward or directorate meet its stated values, the standard of patient care, the budget, staffing levels and policies. Other points may be drawn in where the staff are seeking improvements to meet their own values.

Too much heated discussion must be avoided. Take breaks to allow reflection, further gathering of facts or consultation. Do not expect to achieve an agreed solution at the first meeting. Avoid making any promise that cannot be delivered.

Negotiation is a process of give and take. Each side may give ground on issues deemed most important to the other. Persuasion may induce concessions on short-term issues, if long-term ones will later be achieved.

A written record should be kept of what is agreed on each issue with a copy given to the representative to confirm that the record is accurate.

At the final negotiating meeting, record the changes that have been agreed, together with the date for implementation and a programme for informing all the staff who will be affected by the change. Present it as a joint achievement. Never boast about winning. Fights may be won or lost; in negotiation both sides should have gained some ground.

Further reading

Beare, P.G. (1989) The essentials of win–win negotiation for the Clinical Nurse Specialist. *Clinical Nurse Specialist*, **3**, 3, 138–41.

O

OBJECTIVES – TEAM

Objectives should be simple and precise. They should be developed by the directorate or team leaders of a ward, referring back to the statement of beliefs/philosophy and values to ensure consistency. The mission statement should be reviewed to confirm that the objectives will help achieve it.

Objectives must be expressed in observable or measurable terms, so that progress can be readily identified. Avoid generalized, woolly phrases. Keep them SMART:

Simple;
Measurable;
Achievable;
Relevant;
Timely.

An annual 'away day' can be held to plan the objectives in improving quality. A location where there are no interruptions and from which it is not possible to 'pop back' to work will help everyone concentrate. An allocation may need to be planned within the annual budget to cover 1 day's salaries or bank, agency or locum replacements in order that all the relevant clinical staff can attend. It underlines the message that quality is important.

Each objective will require an action plan and the relevant component agreed and incorporated into each member's performance list. The team objectives can be pinned up by each telephone to remind members of their intentions.

The manager should confirm that the resources will match these plans by checking the strategy and budget for the coming year. At the monthly quality meetings, each action plan should be checked to confirm it is moving the team towards its objectives. If there is no movement, then the relevance of the action plan should be questioned.

OUTSIDE VIEW

An honest outsider's objective view of the quality of a service can be very useful. The manager may be able to ask a respected colleague to visit the directorate once every 3 months and provide a short report of the experience. The visit should be timed for the manager's absence and an outline provided of any changes the team has been trying to achieve. The outsider should be able to speak with the staff and patients to get their views.

The report should be the main item on the agenda of the next quality meeting. The staff should be allowed to correct factual errors. The outside feedback should be used to plan the next area for quality improvement.

The exercise should be repeated by the same outsider so that knowledge of the setting and relationships with the staff are built up.

The directorate should be prepared to provide the same outsiders assessment for others. It provides a useful learning opportunity and enables staff to return and look at their own area with fresh eyes.

P

PETS

Budgies can be boring, you cannot stroke a fish on your lap and cats can be fussy with their favours. Pets are therapeutic, particularly in long-stay settings but more creativity is required in their use.

Animals are very important to some people, sometimes as important as humans. Watching and stroking an animal can be relaxing and reduce stress – except in the phobic! Animals provide something to talk to, to talk about, to care for and a reminder of home. They can enable the demonstration of good feelings, which may not be easy to express. Pets give love and attention and do not ask for much in return. They add to the quality of life.

Arrange for pets to visit their owners. An animal can be a better visitor than some humans: they do not stay too long or upstage a hospital experience with one of their own! A guide dog with its blind owner aids independence and saves the staff time in later rehabilitation. However, staff must check that no other patients nearby are allergic or frightened of the animal.

The following points should be borne in mind when introducing an animal as part of the permanent ward team. Ask the patients and staff for their view on the choice of species. Make a list of the advantages and disadvantages of the ones under consideration; for example, a guinea pig does not usually bite, has clean habits, dry droppings, can be confined to a hutch and is too big to get lost behind cupboards. When required it will sit on a lap for a stroke or snooze. The disadvantages are that the hutch has to be secure, warm, well-ventilated and cleaned out regularly.

Choose an animal with care, arrange an initial health check with a veterinary surgeon and plan for regular check-ups. Get advice on diet, exercise, bedding and hygiene. Buy a reference book on pet care. Put the pet on the payroll or allocate a budget code.

Find a volunteer from among the staff or patients to take responsibility for the animal's overall welfare. Hold a competition to choose a name or draw it from a hat of suggestions.

Unkindness to animals is not easily forgiven. Avoid stress and disputes among staff or patients, and even subtle victimization if someone deliberately hurts the ward pet. Any member of the staff who dislikes the animal should be allowed to avoid situations where this might be evident. If a patient seeks to hurt the pet, staff will need to be vigilant and remove the animal to a temporary place of safety.

If there are problems about having a pet as part of the ward therapy team, consider the PAT (Pro-dog Active Therapy) dogs. Regular visits can be arranged through your local branch.

Quality in practice

Jenny, a teenage girl with paraplegia, had been admitted to a trauma ward. She was withdrawn and no amount of counselling or distraction worked.

The nursing officer's daughter had just acquired a very round, black and white, unfriendly kitten, called George.

He had four white paws and a white spot in an very embarrassing place. He was also very aggressive: he spat if watched and disliked being picked up. He did not have a very pleasant nature.

In those days there was a rule of no animals inside the hospital. The nursing officer, in collusion with the charge nurse, took George, spitting in a sports bag, into the hospital. The screen was around Jenny's bed – she turned her head away and did not respond to the greeting. George was tipped out of the bag onto the bed. He stared at Jenny and spat at her. Her eyes lit up as George slowly, with bottom in the air and head down, stalked her. On reaching her face he gently touched her with soft paws and sat back and stared at her. She laughed, he spat, and the nursing officer tried not to cry.

Every evening George visited the ward, still spitting at the indignity of travelling the short journey in a bag. However, he did seem to appreciate the mobiles now hanging over Jenny's bed. George was a very clean kitten and he used to wash Jenny's chin, spitting at her if she giggled but never hurting her. It was difficult to make sure he was not seen by anyone else, as being round and a bit careless, he would fall off the bed.

There was no doubt that George was the trigger that set Jenny on the road to accepting her paraplegia. Twelve years later she is a teacher, happily married and with two cats and a dog. George went on to be a loving cat (well, most of the time).

Further reading

Cusack, O. and Smith, E. (1984) *Pets and the Elderly*, Haworth Press, New York.

Elliot, V. and Milne, D. (1991) Patient's best friend? *Nursing Times*, **87**, 6, 34–35.

Information

PAT Dog Scheme, Rockey Bank, 4 New Road, Ditton, Kent, ME20 6AD.

PHONE CALLS

The telephonists can put callers and your staff into a good or bad mood, depending on how helpful and efficient they choose to be when a call comes in. The quality of the first point of contact for patients and relatives requires close attention.

As a first step, it is worth visiting the switchboard and meeting the staff. An explanation of the layout of the wards in the directorate in relation to the location of telephones, and of the work organization, can help the telephonist to understand why staff may be slow to answer. If former ward patients may need to telephone a ward for advice, the quality of their experience will be enhanced if the telephonists are aware of possible disabilities. Callers to the ear, nose and throat ward may have speech or hearing defects. Medical wards may treat patients who have speech or thought problems following brain damage.

The telephonists may also have useful suggestions for the ward team which would help provide a higher quality service. Where the switchboard is tucked away in the hospital the telephonists will appreciate a Christmas card and invitation to any ward parties.

One quality check is to telephone a ward in the directorate at a busy time of day. Note how long it takes the switchboard to answer and then for the ward to respond. Consider if the telephonist sounds friendly and the person on the ward sounds helpful. A good quality response should be marked by a letter of congratulation to the switchboard supervisor. If the service was poor then the current strategy needs revision. Some hospitals have invested heavily in training courses in customer service for such 'shop window' staff.

Quality in practice

Bill Brown had been very ill for some time. His family was tired and feeling the strain. The whole Brown family were unimpressed with the nursing care and his condition seemed to be deteriorating. He was to be transferred to another ward. Mrs Brown rang the new ward. The nurse answering the 'phone sounded pleasant: she introduced herself and said she was looking after Mr Brown. She went on to explain his condition, the tests he had received, the provisional diagnosis and what treatment had been started. This primary nurse then suggested that Mrs Brown ring back in an hour for more news and added 'If you feel you want to ring early, please do – I will just go and tell your husband that you are on the 'phone. Do you have a message for him?' A couple of minutes later she returned with a message from Mr Brown to his wife.

As a result of the telephone manner and approach of this nurse some of that family's stress was lifted – they felt safer, they had expected health carers to be kind and helpful. Their confidence, reduced by the experiences of the first ward, now lifted. The subsequent telephone calls reflected the beliefs of the ward team – that patients and relatives deserve information, given in a courteous manner, and to be involved in the patient's care.

PICTURE POWER

A photograph will convey more than a written report and it is quicker. Photographs can illustrate the required quality, position or appearance. They can record changes and capture the successes.

A photograph can also help with a patient's communication problems. Examples include sets of pictures of the main meals to match the menus, photographs of the primary nurse and doctor and the patient's relatives for those who have lost the power of speech. The directorate may find it helpful to have a Polaroid camera available for immediate photographs.

Quality in practice

A former operating theatre was used as a temporary haemodialysis unit. It was a high-risk area with a shared machine. It was difficult to staff and a nightmare to keep clean. Reports were ignored and requests for improvements were turned down. However, within days of the top manager receiving photographs of the area, the services were transferred to another local unit.

Further reading

Williams, W. (1990) A photo opportunity. *Nursing Times*, **86**, 9, 32–34.

PILLOWS

There has not been a hospital ward yet that did not run out of pillows at some point. They fly like 'moths to a light' towards the operating theatre, the accident and emergency department and the laundry.

Arrange a regular visit to the laundry to collect pillows. It gives the laundry staff more space, keeps the cost of replacements down and provides an opportunity for the staff to meet those who toil on their behalf to keep the patients in clean sheets and pillow cases.

PROMISES

Keep them. If asked when a report or change can be delivered, request time to think. Work out how long it will take. If it

requires research, double the time or build in a margin of safety.
Name the date. Deliver early.

The promise of an admission is one that must be kept.
Admission dates for patients should be realistic, taking into
account the likely number of emergency cases that will need
beds. Avoid overbooking. Suggest surgeons keep a separate list
of patients who are willing to come in for operation under local
anaesthetic at very short notice. Call them to fill gaps when there
are more beds free than anticipated. The elderly, retired or unem-
ployed who stay at home and who own a telephone can be easier
to contact. Another option is the loan of a portable telephone so
patients can be contacted at any location. The freelance business
man or woman with a car 'phone and flexibility with deadlines,
such as authors, may be other candidates.

Most patients need to make arrangements with employers,
family or friends to enable them to come into hospital. Several
weeks notice of the date for surgery not only helps the patient
plan, it may also make an uncomfortable condition more toler-
able because a definite end is in sight.

Ask patients to confirm by telephone that they will be attending.
Consider holding a pre-admission clinic to answer questions,
advise on home arrangements for later discharge and save time by
getting tests performed so the results are in the ward for the
patient's arrival.

PUBLIC RELATIONS

Every single member of the staff is part of the public relations
team. In every contact there are opportunities for presenting
the positive aspects of the service and for keeping people
informed.

The manager should use the local system to notify the press
of fund-raising efforts, gifts to the wards, new developments,
the arrival of new equipment, and staff achievements such as
scholarships, awards, publications and promotions. Each hospital has at least one formal contact point for the media. Their help
should be sought in preparing press-releases and in using the
agreed channels to avoid embarrassment to the organization.

Staff have an individual professional responsibility to protect
patients' confidentiality. Written permission must be obtained

before any patient is photographed, even in the background. Great care must be taken if a journalist is invited to observe the work of a ward or department. Mutual trust and rapport can produce real benefits. The 1990 health visitors week was one good example with local papers featuring the work of individual health visitors at the same time as the national press and television covered the profession's activities.

Journalists welcome well-written copy that requires little editing as it can be used to fill an unexpected gap. It should be kept short and snappy. If it requires a lot of rewriting or trimming it may not be used. The 'silly season' in the summer, when there is less political activity, is the time for longer items.

The same item should not be sent to every paper unless it is a 'bare bones', factual news item. The style and readership of a paper or magazine should be noted and the material targeted accordingly. The item should be tailored to the readership; for example, featuring a local firm for the paper's circulation area.

The directorate could consider holding an open day with others to demonstrate equipment and work. A class at a local school could be 'adopted' as a two-way arrangement; a visit to the ward in exchange for a design for the directorate's Christmas card or a display.

Quality in practice

For the Florence Nightingale Commemoration Day, a local primary-school class provided large cardboard models of Florence and a modern nurse. These were placed in the main hospital entrance. Oh to see yourself as children see you – dangling earrings, long hair and bright red nails. The presentation in uniform improved right away.

In return the children visited a ward, the accident and emergency department and the house, in the hospital grounds, where Florence once stayed with her aunt.

Further reading

White, R. (1988) *Advertising: What It Is and How to Do It*, 2nd edn., McGraw-Hill, London.

Q

QUALITY

An activity may have many different qualities. Their relative importance depends on the perception of the recipient. Quality can also be used to denote excellence.

In health care where the service is constrained by the volume of available resources, it may be more useful to indicate whether high quality is to be achieved or a service of adequate quality without the additional expenditure required for the high quality. Precise descriptions of the standard to be provided allows the purchasers and providers to discuss what is desired and achievable. This may not be what the consumers of the service desire.

Poor-quality health services carry risks to life and health. Its delivery may be insensitive or even inhuman.

QUALITY CIRCLES

Quality circles are groups of people, often structured on normal work groups, who meet on a voluntary basis, together with their direct supervisor, to discuss improvements in the current process or better ways of doing things. A facilitator may act as an external resource assisting the group to understand the techniques of problem-solving and group dynamics.

Quality circles can work wonders but there are some ground rules: the leader needs training and the circle needs freedom and space in which to meet. Each member of the group has an equal status within the circle when it is at work. Medical members may find this hard to accept. Domestic and support workers enjoy the change.

Membership is voluntary; a group of up to seven people works best. Meetings should be regular and kept to time. The first steps focus on getting to know each other and in agreeing the general areas to be considered by the group.

The circle needs to find its own identity: tee shirts with a logo are cheap and fun, baseball caps or badges are alternatives. However, they may also be embarrassing to some members.

The group should be asked to select one topic on which to practise the techniques. Brainstorm for as many ideas as come to mind in the given time. The leader should encourage participation no matter how absurd or wild the ideas may seem. No discussion or comment on a particular idea should be allowed during this first flush of ideas. They can be listed in large letters on a flip-chart. The group then takes a short break before discussing all the ideas and seeking links and themes among them. The main ones can then be listed in priority order for practicality. The easiest ideas should be tried out first.

A similar technique may be adopted by a manager who has achieved a good rapport with staff. The facilitator's training course can provide new insights into group work and personal management styles. It may be more appropriate for a manager to act as a facilitator in another directorate rather than try to do so for those being managed.

Further reading

Department of Trade and Industry (1988) *Quality Circles*, DTI, 66–74 Victoria Street, London, SW1E 6SW.

Hyde, P. (1984) *Implementing Quality Circles*, North Warwickshire Health Authority.

Robson, M. (1982) *Quality Circles; A Practical Guide*, Gower, Aldershot.

Robson, M. (1984) *Quality Circles in Action*, Gower, Aldershot.

R

RECRUITING STAFF

Aim to get the best people for the job and to retain them in the organization by developing their skills. High-quality staff support helps recruitment.

Review the recruitment package that is offered. Consider if better crèche facilities, school holiday play schemes, job sharing schemes, discounts from local sports facilities and entertainments would help. Would local housing associations or estate agents offer a special deal for staff? Review the quality and availability of temporary accommodation.

Provide all the information about the post and locality in a smart folder. Local authorities may provide free leaflets on local museums, libraries and beauty spots.

Training costs money. It is a false economy to deliberately recruit those at the lowest incremental point of a salary scale. Quality, in part, depends on knowledge and experience.

The shortlisting and interview panel should consist of two or three people including the immediate manager for the post. Prepare a list of the essential and the desirable knowledge, skills and experience required for the post. Set it alongside a blank column for comments on whether each item is demonstrated by the candidate. Provide each of the panel with a copy for the short listing. It then automatically provides evidence for equal opportunities' monitoring.

Write for references for those shortlisted. Write to the unsuccessful candidates.

The personnel department may offer help with the paperwork involved in recruitment. The staff will also be involved in monitoring for fair practices in recruitment. They will be able to provide information on current pay and conditions of service entitlement for the post.

Ask the panel to meet before the interview to agree the questions to be asked of candidates. Use the list of essential and desirable qualities as a guide. Write down the main questions so that they will be expressed in the same way for each candidate. During the interview this will help compare the candidates' response. Include questions that will assess whether the candidates share the directorate's beliefs and values about quality care and treatment.

Having seen all the candidates, go round the panel to share assessments of each candidate. Managers should be aware that some doctors still tend towards assessments, which are unacceptable in equal opportunities' terms.

Divide the candidates into the clearly unsuitable and the possibles. Examine the references and make a choice. Consider if any of the unsuccessful candidates have the potential for some other vacant post or one that will shortly be vacated. Offer candidates the chance to discuss their interview performance with one or more of the panel, either face to face or later over the telephone.

Interviews can be useful opportunities for staff development and provide a showcase for the directorate. 'Word of mouth' is an effective marketing tool. A positive experience for an unsuccessful candidate may colour their views and help advertise what the directorate has to offer. A poor quality experience may be related in negative terms.

REPORTS

A report conveys information about the year's quality activities. The results give the impression of the last year's strategy and its implementation. It then provides a starting point for planning the next one. The ideal reader or listener wants information that will extend knowledge and, when necessary, help to reach a decision. Managers tend to be inundated with papers.

Rapid reading of reports

Check the title and contents list to confirm relevance. Read the summary and, if still interested, the recommendations. Select those parts of the main body of the text that may yield additional useful information.

Planning to write a report

Consider the purpose of the report and target readership as this will influence the content and the style. A formal research report would follow the conventional scientific format. A report on quality will need to be logical but may be less rigid and illustrated with case studies.

When planning the content, list the topics, sort the information, simplify it and draft the report; then *precis* (summarize) it ruthlessly. Eliminate pontification as facts carry more weight than opinion. Read the draft for ambiguity. Graphs, diagrams and cartoons can convey a meaning more effectively than prose. Use the appendix for details that will only interest a small section of the audience. Keep the report as short and concise as possible.

Core format for reports

These are:

- title page with author's name and date;
- acknowledgements of help received;
- contents list;
- a one-page summary of the key points;
- introduction with the purpose and objectives;
- text giving context, methods, findings and general conclusions;
- recommendations;
- reference list (never plagiarize the work of others);
- bibliography for those who may need to read more broadly about the subject;
- glossary of terms if it is a technical or new subject;
- appendices.

Quality in presentation

The use of graphs, diagrams and photographs to break up the solid blocks of text can make the report easier to follow. A smart cover is worthwhile but shiny paper, pale colours and fancy or small print should be avoided as they make reading uncomfortable. Desk-top publishing packages can be used to turn material prepared on a word processor into an attractive publication.

Distribution

Make reports on quality available to the Community Health Council, any relevant pressure groups and purchasers. Produce a *resumé* for the directorate or hospital newsletter.

Clinical reports

Clinical reports should be accurate, concise, legible, complete and confidential. The Health Service Commissioner (Ombudsman) has been critical of the quality of nursing records.

Managers have a responsibility to ensure that the records system is organized in such a way that confidentiality is maintained. Access to third parties not directly involved in the clinical care must have the patient's informed consent. Computer-based record systems require careful monitoring to ensure any electronic transfer of patient data conforms to this requirement. Data may need to be encoded before transfer via the telephone system so only those authorized to use the decoder will have access to the content.

Patients are entitled to access to their own clinical reports; many directorates aim to share clinical records with the patient. This means that the content must not contain derogatory comments about the patient.

Clinical audit of patient records should include regular audits of the quality of the recording, its breadth and depth. Changes in the layout of standard forms may assist in the completion of reports.

Verbal reports on patients

Verbal reports, like written ones, should be clear, accurate and succinct. Confidentiality is important and the location and involvement of the patient need to be considered. The walking-round report may allow others to overhear personal information.

Courteous involvement of the patient in the discussion of progress can be very effective in increasing the quality of the care provided and in increasing the patient's satisfaction with the process. This means jargon and abbreviations have to be avoided.

Further reading

Calnan, J.R. (1973) *Writing Medical Papers: A Practical Guide*, Heinemann, Oxford.

Calnan J. and Marks, B. (1983) *How to Speak and Write: A Practical Guide for Nurses*, Heinemann, Oxford.

Epitomes and reports from the Health Service Commissioner are distributed to the NHS at intervals. They are also available from HMSO.

Kings Fund Centre (1979) *A Handbook for Nurse to Nurse Reporting*, Project Paper, Kings Fund Centre, London.

UKCC (1993) *Standards for Records and Record Keeping*, UK Central Council for Nursing, Midwifery and Health Visiting, London.

REPRESENTATIVES – COMMERCIAL

Commercial representatives should not be allowed to visit wards and departments unless invited to:

- listen to ideas the staff have for improving one of their products;
- provide teaching sessions on the correct use of their products (see **Equipment – control**).

The worst representatives set out to sell their product at any cost. The best constantly strive to improve their product or to devise a new one to solve the customer's problem. The ones in between will waste staff time.

The good ones treat the staff as honorary consultants for their product. They supply copies of the latest research reports relevant to the clinical area, including bad reviews of their product's performance. The manager should be alert to the amount of time staff spend with such representatives as staff time may be taken away from direct patient care.

REPRESENTATIVES – UNIONS AND STAFF ASSOCIATIONS

Active membership by staff can provide them with extra opportunities to learn new skills such as chairing meetings, keeping minutes and writing reports.

The manager should get to know the local representatives as people with a job to do. The initial assumption should be that they and their members care about the quality of the service offered to patients, even when it is through support departments.

If the directorate's ideas for improving quality will affect other departments or wards, the manager should contact the relevant union representatives to explain what the team proposes to do. That way they can advise their members of the facts if rumours start to circulate.

A further meeting should be promised for when the plans have been drawn up. The ideas and suggestions of the union officers can be helpful. Some are backed by research departments and have access to data that it may be hard to find locally. Suggest the representative shares such information with the team.

If a union representative is a member of the directorate, the manager should keep a record of the time taken off for union duties. If the hospital and the union require increasing amounts of time affecting ward work, the data can be used to press for either temporary replacement hours, or for that person to become a salaried steward and replaced.

Some hospitals and unions have agreed to share the funding of a post because the contribution of an effective steward assists both parties and smoothes the way for improvements and change.

RESISTANCE

Resistance to change is common if preparation is not thorough. Study change theory and be aware of the **honeymoon period.** An unannounced change will throw the staff off balance and they may resist from surprise. Usurping an area the staff thought as their area of responsibility leads to resistance in order to define territory.

Overt opposition stimulates discussion by the team of facts, views and feelings. The manager should listen to both the spoken and the unspoken implications of what is said. The staff may be right. Modification of the proposed change may be sensible.

Avoid attacking one individual. Commitment to one stance means defining the issue and attitudes towards it. Strong attacks will just increase the strength of the opposition. Emotion takes over from cool analysis on both sides.

Try dividing the big issue into a series of small ones. The salami-slicing technique. Chew over the facts for each small issue and gain commitment to it before moving on to the next issue. Once a person publicly agrees to start doing something, it will be more difficult for him to offer a satisfactory excuse for not continuing to do it.

Give the habitual grumbler or disruptive member a specific responsibility for part of the change. They may just be seeking involvement or recognition.

Sabotage by undermining the change through covert action may be hard to spot. Once identified, the manager should marshal the facts and confront those involved to bring the opposition into the open so it can be dealt with as above.

Passive resistance by withholding support is more difficult as it may be denied or even unconscious, such as forgetting to carry out a promised activity by the due date. It may stem from lack of understanding of what is intended, or a lack of commitment to the change.

Sometimes it is necessary for a manager to resist the imposition of an excessive workload on the team. Collect the facts and, if there is time, put them in writing. Inform the team so there is unity of purpose. Emotive wording should be avoided and views presented clearly and calmly. Be aware that the 'foot in the door' of a small compromise can lead to a sequence of commitments which can add up to a major change in workload.

A manager faced with an unacceptable change imposed from above should arrange to discuss the situation with the senior manager. It may also be appropriate to discuss it with the professional organization or trade-union representative. The manager should weigh up the consequences of imposing the change and consider their contribution to the team if they stayed in post or left the organization. Self-respect, integrity and commitment may be at stake. The final decision is a personal one.

Quality in practice

A cardiology consultant obtained the promise of a central monitoring console from a pharmaceutical company and wished to install it at the nurses' station in one ward. A meeting was called, chaired by the operational services manager, involving the sisters from the two cardiology wards, their managers, the consultant and the works officer.

The sisters felt that the change would affect adversely their development of individualized patient care. They also wished to continue to care for their patients in single-sex wards, rather than a one mixed-sex bay. The manager quoted evidence of the additional hours of nurse time required to site a qualified nurse at the console throughout the day and night. There was no money for this.

An alternative plan was proposed: small monitors above each bed and a satellite monitor in the corridor above the nurses' station. This would allow the day staff to observe the tracings as they moved along the corridor and for the monitor to face the nurses' station at night. The staff offered to raise funds for a similar set-up in the second ward if the trial proved successful. The works officer agreed to cost the plan. The meeting broke up with the consultant very resentful at the staffs' resistance to his idea.

An hour later the consultant returned to see the operational services manager. He asked him to ignore the new plan and to place the order for the console so it would be a *'fait accompli'*. Fortunately the manager had recently completed an assertiveness training course and firmly resisted this attempt at sabotage. The alternative plan went ahead and proved a great success.

Further reading

Havelock, R. (1973) *The Change Agents Guide to Innovation in Education*, Educational Technology Publications, New York.
Janis, I.L. and Mann, L. (1977) *Decision Making*, Macmillan, London.

RESOURCE MANAGEMENT

In order to make the most cost-effective use of resources it is vital to be able to monitor their use and be able to adapt and manage in real time. Resource management (RM) requires accurate, timely information in order that the alternative courses of action can be weighed and a decision made by the manager.

Health care is complex and computers help gather data and present information. Access to a personal computer a few hours a week can be very helpful. The manager may be able to arrange this with the management accountant in return for work on areas of mutual interest.

The Department of Health funded NHS hospitals to develop and install information technology to support resource management. The exercise included preparing a detailed project plan and identifying the nature of the information required, with the data needed to produce it. The manager has to assess the need for expert support, training packages and temporary replacement hours to free staff for training. The Information Management Group have produced a wide range of booklets and guidance

notes to help the NHS get the maximum benefit from the investment. (See **Computers.**)

Managers should be cautious about pressure from the finance
department to adopt 'Diagnostic Related Groups' (DRGs), which
were introduced from the USA and modified for use in the UK.
In the USA these were used to set the amount of money paid for
a patient's admission; however, used on their own they failed to
take into account the variations in how ill a patient might be, the
hours of nursing care required, its complexity and the time
needed to deal with the other diseases and disabilities experienced by the patient. Case-mix management systems should be
examined critically for similar weaknesses. Critical-path analyses
or clinical care priorities may offer a more sensitive approach to
calculating the resource use by individuals.

The current nurse-management systems linked to patient care
and dependency calculations require further development before
the estimates of the required nursing resource are reliable and
able to reflect the psychological care and patient education
components. The changes in grade-mix and skill-mix and their
effect on the quality of care require validation before true costs
can be calculated.

Resource management does not depend on computers,
although the technology can help in dealing with large quantities
of data. A manager can seek ways to improve quality by using
the same resources more effectively, or get more of the same
good quality care and treatment from the same resources by
using them in a slightly different way. Hospitals tend to collect a
mass of data that is not used. A little thought can extract useful
information or help make the decision to stop collecting specific
data items. (See **Stopping things.**)

The wise manager makes a friend of the clinical coders who
currently transform the medical diagnoses into international
codes. They can usually be found tucked away in a backroom in
the medical records department. Where patient information is
held on computer, some of the newer systems can automatically
code most of the data. The directorate should be asking for a
printout from the patient administration system (PAS) of the
length of stay by selected primary and secondary diagnoses for
patients admitted over the last full year.

One example might be the use of graduated compression
stockings during and after a specific operation and the occurrence

of deep-vein thrombosis or pulmonary embolism as a secondary diagnosis. In addition, patients re-admitted within 3 weeks of surgery with a primary diagnosis of deep-vein thrombosis will give evidence of whether the rate of DVT is below average. The investment in the stockings can then be judged on whether it gives good value for money.

Another example might be to ask for the pre-operative length of stay. It may be possible to reduce it through the use of a pre-admission clinic to undertake the routine tests. Another solution might be an agreed set of tests performed by the GP with the results sent on to the hospital. The length of pre-operative stay may be reduced if the patient could visit the ward after an outpatients appointment, be given written instructions about 'pre-op' fasting and return to the ward on the day of the surgery, so having a better night's sleep at home.

A copy of the results of any analysis and the changes introduced as a result of the information should be shared with the clinical coders. It can be a lonely working life and they rarely see the patient care results that can flow from later use of the data they patiently entered onto the system.

Quality in practice

In one hospital a detailed study was performed of the resources used by ward attenders who came for blood tests, dressings or to see the doctor. Their data was not being captured on the patient administration system. Senior managers were surprised at this hidden workload and the numbers of needles and syringes, dressing materials, meals and cups of tea and coffee that were used. It solved the mystery of the 'missing' sugar rations. The allocation was based only on the number of inpatients. A separate allocation for the ward attenders was made and this solved a long-standing problem.

Further reading

Munson, P. (1991) Responding to resource management. *Nursing Standard*, **5**, 20.

Resource Management Group (1990) *Collaborative Care Planning*, West Midlands Health Authority, Birmingham.

REWARDS

Performance in any team is distributed along a normal bell-shaped curve. A few outstanding staff at one end, with the bulk of the staff being 'satisfactory' in the middle of the range and a few weaker ones at the other end. Senior managers may reward the outstanding ones on the performance-related pay scheme and make sure the underachievers are not rewarded.

Rewards for team performance can come from celebrations of success, feedback of patient's comments, contributions to the ward/staff amenities fund from copyright, royalties for articles and books (remembering to register books for the public lending right payments) and the sale of teaching packages, the profits from running courses and study days for other health care staff. Rewards for individual performance can come from praise, public acknowledgement (think of the honours list for an example of the pleasure achieved from such a small, national financial outlay), and non-taxable perks such as attendance at a course or study day.

Additional finance may be available to increase the pay of those working in the hard-to-recruit areas of the hospital.

S

SELECTING TOOLS FOR QUALITY MEASUREMENT

In selecting tools for quality measurement, it is important to recognize that some aspects of quality cannot be measured. For these, other quality assessment techniques such as professional opinion or the presence of selected indicators should be considered. It may be helpful to draw up a list of the areas of the directorate's work that could be measured.

Selecting a system to measure quality includes:

- examining the requirements, including time;
- preparing the area and personnel;
- testing the tool or instrument;
- processing the results;
- planning the action based on the results.

The same principles of consultation and discussion should be applied when choosing the system as in all other management procedures. The staff must be involved in the selection as it is their work that is to be measured.

An evaluation of the tools currently available should be undertaken so that the most effective and efficient one is chosen. To do this:

- identify and state what is valued most;
- list the main characteristics to be examined;
- confirm the tool includes these characteristics;
- confirm that measurement is probable;
- decide if the wording of the tool is clear and not open to misinterpretation;
- consider the sources of data are reliable;
- calculate the likely cost of using the tool, analysing the data and interpreting the results.

If the tool fits in with the team's values, is valid, has reliable data sources and is usable, use it with confidence [1].

When first examining quality measuring tools, randomly select some of the standards and/or criteria to check they have the required characteristics.

When considering a commercially available system:

- specify the requirements and invite the firm's consultant or tool designer to explain the system;
- do not be intimidated by the technology or terminology;
- ask to see the system in use in an similar area;
- before observing the system prepare a list of questions;
- talk to the staff where the tool is in use, not just their managers;
- read any available critiques or comments about the system.

Most established systems have workbooks that contain guidelines and research data relevant to the methodology. Some system owners provide a consultancy service; however, the sales talk should be treated with caution. Before purchasing a system, particularly one involving computer software, request the opportunity to run a short pilot test or, if necessary, hire it for a careful review. If the tool proves ineffective it can be discarded with less risk of financial loss.

Occasionally there may be an attempt to impose an unsuitable or untested tool to meet a senior manager's view of what is required. The requirements of the speciality should be described in writing and an explanation of the shortcomings of the proposed tool set out, backed-up by available research.

When a system has been finally selected, it should be tested at intervals of about 1 year for continued validity and reliability. Inter-observer reliability should also be tested. There is a growing literature describing the development and use of quality measurement tools to be found under the 'Quality Assurance' label.

Reference

1. Barnett, D. and Wainwright, P.J. (1987) A measure of quality. *Senior Nurse*, **6**, 3, 8–9.

Further reading

Harvey, G. (1988) Raising standards, the right tools for the job. *Nursing Times*, **84**, 26, 47–48.

Harvey, G. (1988) More tools for the job. *Nursing Times*, **84,** 28, 33.
Kemp, N. and Richardson, E. (1990) *Quality Assurance in Nursing Practice*, Butterworth-Heinemann, Oxford.
McAuliffe, W.E. (1978) Studies of process – outcome correlations in medical care evaluations: a critique. *Medical Care,* **16**, 11, 907–30.

SENIOR COVER

Check that the ward sisters/charge nurses rotate the responsibility to cover for their sickness and annual leave between the senior staff nurses.

Draw up a rota of who will 'act up' as manager for 2–3 months at a time to during any annual leave or sickness or study leave. It should be placed on the ward noticeboards and a copy given to the senior manager and others in the directorate.

The person who is to cover for the manager should be asked to 'shadow' the post for a few days before the first 'acting-up' experience. It should be made clear that the delegated responsibility is total.

The manager should plan his or her leave for the coming year. Regular breaks maintain sensitivity to the actual quality of service being offered. In a well-run team the quality and standard of problem-solving should not dip when the manager is away. It may even go up!

The briefing and debriefing sessions can also be used to seek fresh ideas on the work in hand.

SERVICES

Each service should have its own specified quality standards, particularly if the work is done under an external contract.

If there is a problem that a supervisor has been requested to solve and has failed to act, go to the top manager for that service. Avoid using an intermediary. If it is a long-standing problem or a serious one, arrange a face-to-face meeting.

The manager should agree with the service manager or supervisor which member of their team will act as a designated contact: to be informed of changes within a ward or the directorate, of new ideas for improving quality, and to get to know the particular difficulties that the patients experience because of their health problems.

Keep a list of the contacts, one for each service in each ward information file. Key services that have a direct effect on the quality of care received by patients are:

- catering;
- computing;
- clinical records;
- domestic;
- information;
- laundry;
- pharmacy;
- portering.

Improving the quality of support and clinical services is a two-way activity. The manager can pair one member of the directorate with the designated service contact. The duo can then be asked to work together on reviewing the service received by the ward or directorate and identify any problems the ward staff create for the staff in the support service. Ideas to help staff start this process include the following:

- **Catering**
  Consider the meals provided for patients;
  Review the table and tray settings for ideas to improve the presentation of food;
  Carry out an opinion survey of patients on the choice of meal components, timing, presentation and portion size;
  A list of dates for the food-handlers' course may be used to ensure all permanent staff gain the certificate.
- **Computing**
  Review the training programme for staff at ward level;
  Identify the content of new programmes to increase the opportunities for staff to collect information on their work;
  Examine the record of calls to the computer 'help desk' to identify any common themes from the directorate – consider whether a ward contributed to its own difficulties;
  Confirm the passwords and security codes are not being abused.
- **Clinical records**
  Review the speed with which notes are returned for filing;
  Check whether case files are complete on return or if a

steady trickle of lab. reports follow, so that the records staff
face repeated searching and filing;

Monitor whether the appointment requests are made at
appropriate times of day or whether they are left until they
become 'urgent' and need special attention.

- **Domestic**

    Participation in regular check visits for the cleanliness of
    the area will help identify furniture, fixtures and fittings
    that need replacement or repair. Improvements may reduce
    or speed up the work of the domestic staff;

    Examine the timetable for cleaning, to consider if a change
    in order would enable patients to use the day room for
    breakfast or the bathrooms at more convenient times.

- **Information**

    Review whether all the data required for management
    reports is entered accurately by ward and departmental
    staff;

    Review the range of reports currently requested by the
    ward; do any sit and gather dust?

    Consider whether the staff receive all the useful informa-
    tion obtainable from the data they input to the system.

- **Laundry**

    Consider each ward's record on checking laundry for
    sharps and other objects. If the laundry staff have to spend
    less time checking the dirty laundry they can switch
    resources to the finish achieved for patient clothing and
    linen;

    Consider preparing a 'black museum' of objects retrieved
    from the ward's dirty laundry (a photograph of the
    collected objects placed by the laundry skips in the sluice
    may suffice). Regular updating can reflect improvements.

- **Pharmacy**

    Confirm the stock lists are up to date;

    Review whether the ward pharmacist's skills are fully used
    by staff and inpatient care;

    Consider the place of self-administration in the patient
    care offered in the directorate;

    Review the number and condition of syringe-drivers and
    volumetric pumps in use in each ward; are there enough to
    offer continuous analgesia infusions to all who might need
    them?

- **Portering**
  Are there enough knee blankets available to prevent chilling?
  Does each patient have their own blanket for hygienic
  reasons?
  Do the porters feel confident of their knowledge to prevent
  cross-infection?
  Examine the patient trolleys for rail height to confirm they
  are high enough to contain obese patients safely;
  Check the mattresses on patient trolleys for wear and
  consider whether pressure-relieving pads would improve
  patient comfort.

The manager should ensure there are slots within quality meetings
so that ideas can be shared and improvements celebrated. Useful
changes should be recorded formally so that they can be considered for inclusion in quality specifications, contracts and reports.

SIMPLIFICATION

Examine procedures and instructions, simplify, cut out the frills
or 'what to do if a rare event occurs' sections.

Clarity and the use of simple, plain language in all written
communications will emphasize that enabling all users and staff
to understand and participate is a highly valued quality.

True mastery of a subject is demonstrated by being able to
explain and illustrate the idea so that a student can grasp the core
components, no matter how complex.

SKILL MIX

Skill mix is not the same as staff mix, although they are related.
Examine the skills required from staff by patients, based on the
care and treatment plans.

Staff of different disciplines may have the same skills but at
different stages of development, informed by different depths of
knowledge. They may also use them for different clinical reasons,
based on the particular perspective of each discipline.

Consider whether technology could substitute for some staff
time. Examples include:

- routine pre-operative breathing exercises supervised by the
  physiotherapist may be replaced by use of a respiratory

exerciser of three coloured balls raised in three chambers to be raised by sustained inspiration of air;
- low air loss beds can reduce the need to turn or move heavy patients requiring three or more staff for the procedure;
- automatic peritoneal dialysis machines can free a qualified nurse from 'specialing' a patient.

Activity analysis can be helpful but the observer will only see the physical task, not the mental assessment, interpretation and decision-making processes. This can lead to undervaluing some activities.

When assessing skill mix, identify whether each activity should be performed by a student or support worker at a particular stage of training, or by a qualified person. The more skilled person may undertake other covert activities at the same time. Hunt [1] identified three elements of this multi-functioning:

- **Masking:** for example to make the bed in order to assess the condition of a surgical patient out of bed for the first time;
- **Multi-tasking:** for example assisting a patient to bathe in order to be able to counsel in the privacy of the bathroom;
- **Substituting:** where a non-demanding task is used to relieve stress or to gain thinking time.

Jean Ball and colleagues [2] used a quality assurance tool (Monitor) and a nationwide survey of the different roles of each grade to provide a database for skill mix. This should be considered in the light of the work by Bell and Storey [3] on the skills learnt by each stage of student nurse training, and the relationship to the registered nurse's skills expressed as a percentage. The support worker contribution to patient care and skill level will also vary and needs to be clearly defined in a similar way.

GRASP-type methodology [4] can be used to calculate the hours of nursing care required by patients, based on the actual care plans, divided between the different periods of each day.

If the duty roster is divided into the same periods and the hours of available nurse time are converted into the skill-level percentages, it becomes apparent that the fluctuations in skill level are often out of sequence with the patient requirements.

A similar assessment may be carried out for other health care disciplines.

Improvements can be achieved through flexing shift times, employing part-time and bank staff to assist with sudden peaks in the staff hours required and in adjustments to the skill mix.

The hours of care required by a patient will vary from shift to shift, and from day to day. Managers should seek to invest the resource management money in a system which will record the care plans and automatically calculate the available hours and skill levels required and available. The predicted shortfall or excess allows adjustments before a shift commences. The results can be collected and used to influence the patient admission patterns so that patients receive high-quality care because the staff time available matches the patient hours required.

References

1. Hunt, J. (1990) The activity balance. *Nursing Standard*, **4**, 42, 47.
2. Ball, J., Hurst, K., Booth, M. and Franklin, R. (1989) *But Who Will Make the Beds? A Research-based Strategy for Determining Nursing Skill Mix for the 1990s*, The Nuffield Institute and Mersey RHA, Leeds University, Leeds.
3. Storey, C. and Bell, A. (1985) A useful pair of hands? *Nursing Times*, **81, March 27**, 13, 40–42.
4. Milne, C. (1988) Getting to grips with GRASP. *Nursing Standard*, **3**, 22–23.

STAFF MIX

The mix of staff from different disciplines available to provide patient care and service forms an important resource for delivering high-quality service. Consider the extent of the range of skills offered by each of the disciplines, based on their professional education and from on-the-job training.

Ward clerks and domestic staff also form an important part of the ward team, with phlebotomists and technicians assisting the doctors with the medical workload of blood sampling and physiological measurements. In wards for the elderly, the patients' fluid intake may depend on the domestic staffs' interest in matching the container to each patient's needs and even helping them to drink.

Inevitably it is in the 'grey area' of overlapping skills and knowledge that expensive time can be released for other professional activities. Repetitive care and treatment that can be well-defined and is not associated with covert assessment and decision-making may be suitable for transfer to another discipline. This usually only works in non-acute settings where the patient's clinical condition is stable.

When the other discipline needs repeated instruction or has to call on the professional for decisions it reduces the total hours available for patient care, as two people are needed: one of whom may be unable to undertake other work while waiting for the other to finish a task.

Thus it is often more cost-effective and delivers higher quality care to have a high proportion or all-qualified nurse team rather than rely on a small proportion instructing and supervising an army of nursing assistants. The less-qualified will have a lot more 'down time' compared with the qualified nurse. The budget pays for this time lost from direct patient care.

Within a discipline, the grade mix may vary according to the patient group. The mix of enrolled and registered nurses is slowly swinging towards more registered nurses. There are also variations between general nursing, paediatrics, mental illness and mental handicap.

Be aware that the Department of Health's report 'Mix and Match' [1] confuses skill mix with staff mix. Its conclusions are considered by many to be unsound [2].

There is a relationship between the number of staff required and the size of the ward. Small wards require a higher number of hours per patient because of the need for safety cover, particularly at night.

References

1. Wright-Warren, P. (1986) *Mix and Match*, DHSS, London.
2. Moores, B. (1987) Janforum: Comment on 'Mix and Match': a review of nursing skill mix. *Journal of Advanced Nursing*, **12**, 765–67.

Further reading

Buchan, J. (1990) Paying for performance. Policy notes. *Nursing Standard*, **14**, 21, 44–45.
Buchan, J. (1990) Grade mix. *Nursing Times*, **4**, 34, 54.
Grey, A. (1987) A mixed review. *Senior Nurse*, **6**, 2, 6–8.
Harrison, S. (1990) *The Contribution of Domestic Staff to the Welfare of Mentally Ill In-Patients*, Durham University, Health Care Research Unit, Durham.

STAFF SHORTAGE

The NHS is the largest employer of staff in the UK. However, the Judge Commission [1] found that there will be a reduction in the number of young people available to enter nursing in the 1990s. This would also effect recruitment to the other health professions. The traditional reliance on a steady stream of young people entering health care is being influenced by demographic changes. Some clinical specialities have long-standing problems in attracting and retaining specialist staff, such as nurses in operating theatres, occupational and speech therapists. Management is, in part, about anticipating and planning how to deal with difficult situations; staff shortage is one such situation.

The actual and potential reasons for shortage of staff may include:

- increased workload;
- staff sickness;
- high turnover of staff;
- antisocial hours;
- task-allocated work;
- poor salary compared with others of equal responsibility;
- dull recruitment policies and procedures;
- uninspired continuing educational programmes;
- inappropriate leadership styles.

Salvage [2] suggests:

> Recruitment indicates that the biggest source of returners are women – not in paid employment but taking breaks to raise children. The factors influencing whether they will return include staffing levels, pay, availability of refresher courses, quality of counselling/support and provision of part-time posts. Crèche facilities are also rated highly by many younger nurses.

The solutions to actual and potential staff shortage may include one or more of the following actions:

- **Review reasons for staff leaving**
  Exit interviews are a means of finding out the reason for staff leaving a ward. A questionnaire with a stamped addressed return envelope sent to former staff may also give useful information. However uncomfortable the

findings may be for the manager, action should be taken, where possible, on the results;
'Stay in touch' schemes may also bring results [2];
Examine the research findings on workforce wastage for new ideas or insights.
* **Make working conditions more attractive**
Examine the recruitment policy and change it if necessary;
Cost out a crèche facility and charge a realistic fee; a subsidy may be necessary;
Consider flexi-time and job-sharing;
Assess if the traditional shift system could be changed to a more flexible roster;
Welcome potential bank staff, whatever hours they work.
* **Seek replacement staff**
Support 'Return to work' courses;
Join with other managers to organize an 'open evening or day' for people interested in working in the health service;
Consider assertiveness training for new members of staff;
Listen to the comments of new staff: they often raise issues that those who have been in the hospital for some time no longer notice;
Organize a mentor system for new staff who have had a break from their profession.
* **Make the work more satisfying**
Look at how work is organized and consider enhancing staff responsibility by implementing a professional model of organizing care, for example primary nursing;
Look for outmoded practices;
Liven up the education programme with help from the continuing education department;
Check that part-time and night staff have equal access to staff development and education programmes.
* **Make staff feel valued**
When staff are off sick for any length of time, the manager should demonstrate his or her concern by sending a get-well card, or 'phoning to see how they are, without giving the impression that they are being checked up on;
Recognize the contribution of staff to team work, give feedback on their work [3];
Set up staff-support groups and have access to an independent counsellor.

- **Control the workload**
    Review the workload with the medical staff to see if
    changes in the planned admissions can reduce the work-
    load for staff;
    Use the quality scores and patient-dependency data to bid
    for additional staff to meet the workload;
    Collect factual examples of omissions of care or treatment
    because of the limited staff hours recorded in the nursing
    or other clinical notes;
    Changes in duty rosters should only be made with the
    consent of the staff and consideration of the knock-on
    effects on later shifts;
    Review the workload pattern for peaks and troughs, and
    the staffing profile for the related skill mix for possible
    adjustment to even out the load on individuals;
    Discuss the contracts for possible adjustment with the
    agreement of the purchasers.
- **Plan for emergencies**
    Make contacts with local voluntary organizations prepared
    to help in an emergency;
    Agree a policy on who may close beds to new admissions;
    Prepare a checklist of the steps to be followed to deal with
    surges in workload. Include contact with the medical staff,
    support services, medical records staff, admissions unit,
    and other wards where emergencies will be admitted;
    Budget for the use of bank and agency nurses to cope with
    peaks in workload;
    Clarify the local rules for virement between budgets to
    cope with emergencies.

References

1. Judge commission (1985) *The Education of Nurses: A New Dispensation*,
   Royal College of Nursing, London.
2. Salvage, J. (1989) Whistling in the wind? *Nursing Times*, **84**, 41, 24.
3. Blanchard, K. and Johnson, S. (1985) *The One Minute Manager*,
   Fontana/Collins, Glasgow.

Further reading

Birch J. (1975) *To Nurse or not to Nurse*, Royal College of Nursing,
London.

Clay T. (1987) *Nurses Power and Politics*, Heinemann, London.

Gray, A. and Normand, C. (1990) Hidden costs of turnover. *Health Service Journal*, **100** (5225), **November 1**, 1646–47.

Morton-Cooper, A. (1988) Managing a successful return. *Nursing Times*, **84**, 49, 41–42.

Shepperdson, B. (1990) Clinical recruitment: why nurses leave their jobs. *Nursing Standard*, **4**, 22, 27–30.

Williams, C., Soothill, K. and Barry, K. (1991) Love nursing, hate the job. *Health Service Journal*, **101**, **February 14**, 18–21.

STALE MANAGERS

It may take 4–5 years before the signs start:

- polishing the image, not greasing the wheels of progress;
- sitting only with certain people in the dining room or at meetings;
- short-tempered with honest criticism;
- preoccupied with reducing costs, not how to improve quality;
- months behind on the professional and management reading;
- watching the clock to see if it is time to go home, rather than to check if there is time to fit in another activity;
- avoiding risks;
- staff who hesitate before mentioning something;
- no really new ideas for months.

Burnout can occur in managers. Trying too hard, not taking regular breaks to 'recharge the batteries' and not sharing the load can all take their toll. The more senior the position, the longer it takes to achieve significant changes because the span of influence is so much wider. No wonder some managers give up in the job.

Working in a hierarchy can be difficult if more senior posts are filled by ineffective managers or those who have lost their enthusiasm for the job. Learning how to manage the stale or burntout senior manager becomes essential if progress is not to be impeded. One persistent problem is likely to be delays through a lack of decisions from the stale manager.

The more-junior manager may try preparing a paper on a favourite project, spelling out the problems and the possible answers, with an action plan. Leaving one or two 'easy to spot' gaps for the boss to point out may catch the required interest. If the situation is really difficult it may also be necessary to send a copy to the boss's boss for information. The more-junior manager should also volunteer to make the next move (the monkey of the Oncken monkey management techniques) and offer possible dates to report back on progress (see **Delegation**).

STANDARDS

Standards help the hospital to measure whether it really has put into action its values and beliefs held by staff about the quality of care and treatment of patients. The standard should be a statement of the 'agreed level of performance appropriate to the population addressed' [1].

Each standard may need several measurable criteria. Such descriptive statements cover the behaviour, circumstances or clinical condition of the patient.

Be warned that some inexperienced people misuse the terms 'standards' and 'criteria', causing confusion by using them interchangeably. The confusion may be increased by tools calling criteria 'items' or 'cues' and using 'objectives' for standards. Bloch [2] clarifies the reasons for correct usage. Standards not only identify deficiencies but can then also reinforce good practice and outcomes.

The manager should not waste time and 'reinvent the wheel'. Instead the team can be asked to check that no one else has developed written standards that would suit the field of work. Adapting someone else's tool can give staff a sense of ownership while saving time. Such adaptations should be recorded and the origin of the tool properly acknowledged on any printed version. An adapted tool requires the same validation tests as a new one.

Standard-setting from scratch should be costed. The manager should also consider the stress level it may create for some staff. The final tool can be tailored to local needs. The result can give a sense of pride and ownership, so that it is used and thought useful.

If possible, the manager should use a multi-disciplinary group so that different perspectives can be considered. For patient care and service standards, collect the views of patients. If that is not possible, include a member of the **Community Health Council**, a relevant ginger group or a regular inpatient. The group can consider using a facilitator with a knowledge of quality assurance, teaching and group dynamics. The manager may try to include someone in the group who knows about the relevant research or where to find it. Meetings require a comfortable room where the group will be free of interruptions.

At the start, the group will need facts and guidelines on how to set standards. A workshop setting can provide privacy while practising new skills. A session on group dynamics can help foster tolerance and speed up the group work. A critique of the first efforts by an experienced standards officer may be helpful.

The group should choose subjects that are giving cause for concern or are recent innovations. Select the target population by age, gender, diagnosis, disease or the discipline providing their care. In a homogenous population the standard would be expected to apply to everyone.

The manager should advise the group to pick a framework from among the many described in the literature. It will help to ensure that the 'what?', 'when?', 'where?' and 'why?' of each criterion are not forgotten.

The World Health Organization [3] have set out targets to be met by the year 2000 entitled 'Targets for Health for All'. Some managers are using them in formulating their new contracts. Others see them as a basis for setting standards and auditing.

References

1. RCN (1986) *Standards of Care Project – Checklist on How to Write Standards of Nursing Care*, Royal College of Nursing, London.
2. Bloch, D. (1977) Criteria, standards, norms – critical terms in quality assurance. *Journal of Nursing Administration,* **September**, 20–30.
3. World Health Organization (1984) *Targets for Health for All*, WHO Regional Office for Europe, Copenhagen.

Further reading

Kemp, N. and Richardson, E. (1990) *Quality Assurance in Nursing Practice*, Butterworth-Heinemann, Oxford.
Kendall, H. (1988) Raising the standards: the West Berkshire approach. *Nursing Times*, **84**, 27, 33–34.
Kitson, A. (1990) *Quality Patient Care: The Dynamic Standard Setting System*, Scutari, Harrow.

STOPPING THINGS

It is easier to start a new idea than to stop an old one. Before trying a new activity that will take time to carry out once it is up and running, decide which old activity will be stopped to free up that time.

Once a year the team should hold a brainstorming session to consider whether there are any:

- old beliefs still going strong, such as salt in the bath water, routine TPR measurements, specimens or X-rays that get repeated without a clinical assessment of need;
- out-dated practices such as the use of Eusol for wound cleansing, or liquid paraffin used to stop dressings from adhering to wounds, which actually delay wound healing;
- inefficient tools such as forms or reports that have lost their purpose.

The time saved can be used to enhance the value of activities that can be shown to be effective.

STUDENT NURSES

Clinical areas selected for student-nurse placements are audited once a year by a nurse teacher and a clinical nurse. The audit may be repeated more frequently if a ward is not reaching the required criteria. The number of qualified nurses in an area will determine the maximum number of students who may be allocated there. A hospital also needs to ensure the proper supervision of unqualified staff in order to maintain effective patient care.

The threat of having students withdrawn can be a strong motivator to improve the quality of the learning environment and the quality of care offered to patients. If the qualified nurses respond in a negative way, the manager should look for the reasons and take the appropriate action. A poor learning environment is usually providing poor quality patient care.

The ward sister/charge nurse should be familiar with the student's curriculum and the relevance of the ward learning objectives to the rest of the course. *Project 2000* students are supernumerary during their early placements; in the later stages they need carefully planned increased responsibility for patient care. Semi-structured teaching sessions specifically for students can help integrate the theory with their current clinical experiences.

Assessment of the students' clinical competence is the responsibility of the ward sister/charge nurse and each student's mentor.

Students must be interviewed at the start of the placement to discuss the learning objectives, to establish their specific needs, and to identify their strengths and difficulties. The mentor or ward sister may seek further discussion with the manager, particularly if the student requires extra help.

The student should be interviewed about progress at least once during the middle of the placement. The person conducting the interview should ensure they have enough time, without interruption, to discuss the student's work in a constructive way and to help the student evaluate the quality of the experience.

Allowance should be made for each student's stage of learning. The manager should ensure students are treated correctly and fairly, with duty rotas planned so they can work with their mentors, opportunities to observe and to practise skills, praised for good work and for trying to improve. Constructive criticism should be given when a student errs. The manager should be alert to possible favouritism among the staff, or victimization by those who feel threatened by the intelligent and articulate student who questions current ward practice. The conformist student may also be at risk and the manager needs to be alert for bullying by staff or fellow students. The quality of the experience can be compared with the Royal College of Nursing's Bill of Rights for Students [1].

If a student is unhappy during a ward placement, initially the mentor should deal with the problem. According to Burnard [2] 'Mentors help bridge the theory practice gap ... they inspire and advise.' If the mentor cannot resolve the problem – the mentor may be the problem – then the ward sister or teacher should be involved. The manager may need to be involved if the staff relationship with a student or students is causing a problem, particularly as patients could be drawn into the situation.

Student nurses have a responsibility for their actions and for their behaviour. They should not be over-protected. The manager should confirm that the students know the correct channels for dealing with problems. Apparently kind people can be as culpable as the obviously poor ones: perhaps more so, as they are difficult to spot and, as a result, may do more to damage quality.

Quality in practice

A ward sister who returned to nursing after a career break soon began to have a high level of student sickness on her ward. She could not understand this or find out why; the patient questionnaires praised the staff, and in particular the ward sister's courtesy and kindness to both patients and staff. When she asked the students she received evasive answers and no positive response. The qualified nurses and teachers would not admit anything was wrong.

In desperation the ward sister invited four past students to tea in the ward office. There were no other qualified nurses present. She told them of the problem and her puzzlement. Eventually one of the students explained that the ward was in their opinion the worst of their placements. They complained they were never included in any of the decision-making, they were over-protected and were never allowed to use any initiative. When they had tried to complain to the qualified staff, including a teacher, they had been criticized and the sister's kindness was highlighted.

One student added 'You drove me mad, you insulted us, we are not children, we are adults but no one believed us.' The sister was shocked but thanked the students and apologized saying she would correct the situation for the present students. Sadly as they left the office she heard one say 'Why do I feel so rotten when it isn't me who is in the wrong?'

References

1. RCN *Nursing Students Bill of Rights,* Royal College of Nursing, London.
2. Burnard, P. (1990) Is anyone a mentor? *Nursing Standard,* **4**, 37, 46.

Further reading

Barlow, S. (1991) Nurse education issues – impossible dream. *Nursing Times,* **87**, 1, 53–54.

Fretwell, J. (1982) *Ward Teaching and Learning: Sister and The Learning Environment*, Royal College of Nursing, London.

Fretwell, J. (1985) *Ward Freedom to Change; The Creation of a Ward-learning Environment*, Royal College of Nursing, London.

Ogier, M. and Cameron-Buchari, R. (1990) Supervision: a cross-cultural approach. *Nursing Standard*, 4, 31, 24–25.

Mangan, P. (1990) Bill of rights, clause nine. Tradimus. *Nursing Standard*, 4 (suppl.), 31, 63–64.

Reid, N.G. (1985) *Wards in Chancery? Nurse Training in the Clinical Area*, Royal College of Nursing, London.

SUCCESS

Celebrate success: new ideas, major improvements in a patient's condition or a hard-won minor improvement. A manager is the chief salesperson, extolling the achievements of the team inside and outside the hospital. He or she can do this by:

- telling the press;
- adding a short report in the hospital newsletter;
- having a party after work;
- organizing a celebratory meal, an outing to the local ice rink, bowling alley, burger bar or inn;
- using videotape to record new procedures, operations or equipment;
- displaying photographs with a notice explaining what was achieved and who was involved;
- considering adding a photograph to the information letter to local GPs;
- writing to tell the GPs of the latest innovations.

Celebrating the patients' achievements also helps their motivation.

Prepare an annual report listing the developments and successes; attach it to the strategy for the coming year. The manager should also write on behalf of the directorate to congratulate individuals on examinations passed, publication of articles, reports completed, long service and special contributions to the work of the unit.

T

TEACHERS

Teachers who work in a ward are members of the health care team and must be accepted as such. Medical and nurse teachers should ask the patient's permission to involve him/her in the teaching process. The information booklet for patients should explain the right to refuse to participate.

Teacher-practitioner posts provide joint appointments between hospital and college. University medical staff who teach medical students have held honorary consultants posts for many years. In nursing, the post may be at ward-sister level, or with the teacher acting as a primary nurse to a particular group of patients, perhaps sharing care with student nurses. The advantages of teacher-practitioner posts include:

- the potential for educating the whole ward team;
- acting as a role model and consultant;
- ensuring the classroom teaching is based on up-to-date clinical practice;
- ensuring that ward practice is based on sound theory.

The disadvantages include a conflict of loyalties, a heavy work-load and possible loss of continuity of patient care.

Those teachers in general education who come from outside the health service to teach patients, as in children's wards, must also be treated as part of the ward team.

High quality teaching requires information about the ward, and also adequate resources in a suitable environment. Teachers from all disciplines need an orientation programme and to be given a copy of the ward beliefs. In addition, the general teacher may require an explanation of the different health-service roles and the ward culture; also a brief explanation of the types of conditions patients may be suffering and how this may affect their attention span, and/or their ability to learn.

Ideally, a teaching room should be available in each directorate. If possible buy or borrow equipment. The frequency and quality of teaching sessions may be increased by provision of an over-head projector, flip-chart, pens and other supplies. To ensure that teaching supplies and equipment do not disappear, a strict procedure for using the room should be devised. The teacher(s) who do not have a convenient base should be provided with a locker and key.

The manager can help the teacher to be effective in the ward area by clarifying the working relationship and the chains of communication and by involving the teacher in study days and planned innovations – they can often bring a different perspective to a project. Invite them to coffee breaks and social functions as the ward teacher can feel isolated. Give the teacher feedback on his or her performance. Be alert to signs of stress. It is often presumed that if a person is 'bright' or well-qualified academically they will cope, whatever the situation; this is not always so. Develop an awareness of possible tensions that can occur between colleagues.

The manager and teacher should meet at specific intervals to discuss the teacher's work in the directorate and to identify how the one can help the other. It is necessary to know the times and dates of the teacher's proposed visits to the wards to ensure the teaching programme is incorporated into the planned ward activities.

Further reading

Crane, S. (1989) Joint appointments, the Deakin experience. *Australian Journal of Advanced Nursing*, **6**, 3, 21–25.

Guilbert, J.J. (1987) *Educational Handbook for Health Personnel, (6th edn), WHO Offset Publication No. 35*, World Health Organization, Geneva.

Kemp, N. (1984) *Practitioner Teachers in Quality Assurance Programmes in North America*. Smith and Nephew Florence Nightingale Report, The Florence Nightingale Committee, London.

Kershaw, B. (1990) Clinical credibility and nurse teachers, Supplement 'A Strategy for Nursing'. *Nursing Standard*, **4**, 51 46–47.

Marson, S. (1990) Creating a climate for learning. *Nursing Times*, **86**, 17, 53–55.

Vaughan, B. (1989) Two roles – one job. *Nursing Times*, **85**, 15, 52.

TEMPORARY CLOSURES

Increased flexibility in the use of limited resources now leads to more temporary closures, for example, to make financial savings over holiday periods. Plan well ahead. Include temporary closures in the budget plans. If possible select periods that fit with the local school holidays so staff can have the opportunity to take annual leave while the ward is closed. Staff should not be pressured into taking an unplanned break.

If possible use the opportunity to provide updating or a desired change of clinical experience for staff who choose to work during the closure. Uncertainty can be reduced by arranging the temporary relocation well in advance. This allows staff to visit the new area and get to know the staff with whom they will be working.

The Community Health Council should be informed of the dates for the closure. Confirm with the clinical records department that they have recorded the dates for their bed returns. For some reason the commissioning of wards receives more attention than the temporary closure. A well-planned campaign is better than chaos!

Prepare for the temporary closure by alerting all the service departments and agreeing any prior run-down of stocks. Plan for a review of all the stocks. Any coming close to an expiry date during the closure should be transferred for immediate use elsewhere. Check if routine maintenance can be carried out before any cleaning or decorating is performed during the closure period. Bed curtains may need to be removed for laundering. Consider if there will be enough time to get old bedframes or chairs refurbished. Book such services well in advance.

Confirm that locks and keys are in working order, or contact the works department to arrange for a carpenter to fix a hasp and staple to the doors so they can be padlocked. Alert the fire officer or the health and safety officer in case temporary changes in the evacuation procedure for other areas will be required.

Arrange for the relocation of patients. Provide them with an explanatory letter for relatives and visitors. Put a notice on the ward door to warn of the impending temporary closure.

Make out a checklist room by room of all the arrangements to be completed on the day of the move. Colour code for time or priority order. Photocopy it for future reference. Find the ward inventory.

On the day of the move, people should be the manager's first priority. The patients should be discharged or transferred with all their property and the paperwork completed. Each member of the staff should be allocated specific tasks and responsibilities. The checklist should be ticked off as each activity is completed.

The pharmacist will wish to oversee the return of controlled drugs and the completion of the appropriate records.

Arrange for someone from the hospital administration to go through the inventory with the ward sister and to sign as a witness that a true record of all the equipment has been made. Missing equipment should be noted. Clean and forlorn items get treated as fair game by any light-fingered visitor or inefficient ward. Equipment that looks as if it is organized ready for re-opening discourages theft. Lock the doors and arrange for secure storage of the keys.

Review the checklist for potential improvements and to plan the re-opening process.

Further reading

Pettingell, Y.A. (1988) A ward sister's guide to a ward move, *Nursing*, **3**, 30, 30–35.

TESTING – EQUIPMENT

Novel clinical items may need ethics committee approval if there is any risk to staff or patients.

When new items are to be purchased ask for test reports on reliability, flammability and for the manufacturer's recommendations for servicing. Arrange a demonstration and a trial period. A member of the team should be delegated to co-ordinate the testing period. A standard format should be used to record the staff's comments, their ideas for improvements and any problems in use. Manufacturers concerned about quality appreciate such feedback.

The Department of Health provides a range of technical memoranda and health equipment notices. The comparative and descriptive studies of electromedical and mechanical equipment provide a useful source of ideas; they should be in the hospital library.

Directorates should be cautious about servicing contracts. It may be cheaper to make local arrangements for electromedical and computer equipment rather than send equipment away. Some companies will provide an on-site service or provide temporary replacement equipment.

Cheaper, poor-quality equipment may earn the firm more money from repairs, replacements and servicing than is saved at the original purchase.

Regular inspection and calibration of items such as sphyg-momanometers should be planned so that staff can trust the accuracy of clinical measurements.

Check the speed with which the NHS safety information bulletins and hazard warning notices reach the staff.

Further reading

Norton, D. (1970) *By Accident or Design?* E.S. Livingstone, Edinburgh.
Norton, D. (1986) Measuring product performance. *Professional Nurse*, 2, 3, 81–83.

TOTAL QUALITY MANAGEMENT

The NHS Executive has encouraged hospitals to adopt total quality management (TQM) as a long-term aim; to 'build in quality' to the process of care and treatment.

The culture of the hospital has to change to become patient-centred. This means the outpatient appointment system is designed to minimize the waiting period for the patient rather than for the doctor. It means information leaflets, individual care plans, choice of admission dates and choice of treatment options when available.

To achieve TQM, every aspect of the organization and delivery of patient and diagnostic services, care and treatment is assessed and a programme to improve the quality developed. In a complex organization, such as a hospital, this requires considerable integration of all the strategies and activities involved in managing quality. It includes inspection, quality control of resources, monitoring, audit and quality assurance.

Managers have to facilitate these changes. Commitment from most senior staff is essential. A detailed strategy is required, with the focus on achieving quality and effectiveness considered in planning any changes. The many different components have to slot together and support each other. Education programmes have to be developed and staff released to attend so that the proportion familiar with quality management techniques expands, until the whole place is involved from the most senior consultant to the newest member of the backroom staff.

Patients' expectations are increasing. They look for prompt, efficient, helpful service, particularly from the support services such as catering, portering, reception and clinical records staff in the outpatients department.

Patient satisfaction profiles can be compiled from surveys conducted by the staff, the quality assurance department or with help from the **Community Health Council**. Feeding back the patients' views and the general level of satisfaction, while tackling the individual complaints or comments, provides a major challenge.

Managers also have to support the development of the clinical dimensions of quality by the health care professionals through daily reports of activity, surveys, audits, education and training.

Further reading

Brooks, T. (1992) Total Quality Management in the NHS. *Health Services Management*, **88** (2), **April**, 17–19.

Calman, K.C. (1992) Quality: a view from the centre (setting national standards). *Quality in Healthcare*, **I**, Supplement 28–33.

Colard, R. (1989) *Total Quality: Success Through People*, Institute of Personnel Management, London.

Davies, H. (1992) Role of the Audit Commission. *Quality in Healthcare*, Supplement 36–9.

Freemantle, N. (1992) Spot the flaw. *Health Service Journal*, **102** (9), **July**, 22–24.

Fullerton, H. and Price, C. (1991) Culture change in the NHS. *Personnel Management*, **23** (3) **March**, 50–53.

Morris, B. (1989) Total Quality Management. *International Journal of Health Care Quality Assurance*, **2**, 3, 4–6.

NHS Management Executive (1993) *Achieving an Organisation Wide Approach to Equality*, EL(93)116, Department of Health, Leeds.

Useful source of information

International Journal of Health Care Quality Assurance, published by MCB University Press Ltd, Bradford, England.

U

UNITY

Unity equals harmony and concord between persons.

It means pulling together to achieve a common goal such as high-quality health care. That means the team members must identify common **values** and be willing to compromise on their personal views for the common good.

Unity is necessary when in a difficult situation. It therefore beholds any manager to try to form good relationships, not only for the sake of good team morale but also for survival!

V

VALUABLES

What is of great financial worth may not be a patient's most valued possession. While it is essential that staff record any jewellery, watches, or large sums of money that a patient has brought into hospital with them, the family photographs, letters and even 'get well' cards can mean more to the patient. Taking good care of the patient's possessions demonstrates that staff value the patient.

The wearing of jewellery of great sentimental or religious value may outweigh the risk of loss. Dentures and spectacles (the former often being thrown away with the tissue they were wrapped up in) should always count as valuable.

Some hospital policies are so tight they require staff to take into safe-keeping anything of value whether or not the patient is able to guard their personal property. Such paternalism does not acknowledge the patient's right to be involved in decisions. The manager should review the way the current policy is operated. If the patient will be out of action for a brief time, for example while in the operating theatre, propose a scheme for endorsement of the patient's capability and limited use of the ward safe. If this is agreed, explain the system in the booklet for inpatients.

Check that there are facilities for storing valuables belonging to the patients admitted after office hours.

Check also that the policy for returning the items is sensitive to a patient's needs. Insisting that cash deposited for safe-keeping can only be returned in the form of a cheque is unhelpful and insensitive when the patient has no bank account and is likely to feel too ill or disabled to leave home for several days or weeks. Check the print on receipts is clear and large enough for easy reading by the elderly. Educate the general office administrative staff on the reasons why greater flexibility will enhance the overall quality of service to patients.

Quality in practice

A wealthy elderly woman, admitted to a ward late one evening, had brought her favourite rings. She would only allow the nursing staff to have responsibility for the jewellery that was valued at many thousands of pounds. The nurse in charge of the ward rang the manager, for guidance. The manager was not sure what to do. She returned to the ward and with the nurse in charge found a procedure on 'handling valuables'. At the end of the unhelpful script they read 'If you do not know what to do, approach your manager.' An early review of the ward policy would have spared the manager embarrassment. The staff decided to accept the patient's wishes. They listed the items and placed them in the ward safe. In the morning they were able to arrange with the patient for a trusted relative to collect the majority of the rings for transfer to her local bank. The patient was able, after treatment, to wear her favourite ring for the rest of her hospital stay.

VALUES

Values need to be brought out into the open and discussed. Shared beliefs about health care may be further influenced by different values put on those beliefs. The manager's values drive the vision of high-quality health care.

Health care professionals have strong beliefs about:

Authority
Autonomy
Accountability

They value autonomy and have come to recognize that accountability operationalizes authority.

The reward and recognition system of the hospital should reinforce the highly valued activities. Too often it appears to those working at the bedside that the paperwork is valued more highly than skilled hands-on patient care. The work systems limit autonomy and often site accountability at several levels beyond the action (see **Disobedience**).

The values of each professional group need to be made explicit so that areas of tension or potential conflict can be recognized and explored. Conflict can be healthy and help a hospital to change its policies and procedures.

Patients and their carers may have different values. The pressure group 'Action for Sick Children' has achieved considerable change in the professions' recognition of the value of parental contact during a child's stay in hospital. The parent's contribution is now valued and so encouraged.

VISION

The effective leader holds in his or her head a simple, clear, crisp vision of what the positive outcome will look like.

That vision has to be conveyed to everyone in the team, so that they share the picture and can play their part in achieving the desired quality. Greater autonomy then becomes a natural part of the process as everyone starts to trust their colleagues to work for the same goals.

Think big, start small. Let the team share in the work so it becomes their responsibility too.

The leader who cares passionately about the quality and care offered by the team will create enthusiasm, unity and a desire to achieve technical excellence as well as intense interest in the welfare of patients and their relatives.

People then start looking forward to the day's work.

W

WELCOME

An effective ward or unit carries with it a family feeling. Patients feel they are joining the staff team and see a role in achieving their own recovery.

The feeling of welcome should start at the door: a greeting on entering, introductions to patients and staff. A long wait on arrival can increase fear of the unknown.

The quality team should consider the following:

- a notice of welcome by the door;
- up-to-date magazines in waiting areas;
- a personalized letter or booklet of welcome placed in the patient's locker, with useful information about the ward;
- a list of the names of the staff and a map of the ward or unit;
- flowers, real or imitation, to brighten the room;
- a guided tour of the ward or unit;
- a choice of meal, even if the orders have to be placed 24 hours in advance;
- information about the area for new staff or students attending for clinical experience;
- a letter of welcome to new staff before they arrive.

If the patient is considered an honoured guest, it becomes second nature to use the symbols linked with that status:

- the tray to deliver drinking water and glass, or cup of tea;
- soap and hand-towels always available near the 'loo';
- the ward television or radio only switched on for the patient's entertainment – not the staff's.

WHISTLE BLOWING

The term whistle blowing, in relation to NHS staff raising issues of concern in public, came to prominence in the early 1990s. The introduction of NHS Trusts, as providers of health care, brought with it new freedoms to set local contracts of employment. While the details of individual patients have always had to be kept in confidence there were attempts to add confidentiality clauses about more general activities of the organization.

These were used to try to stop hospital staff reporting serious problems to others outside the hospital. Reductions in staff numbers and in services also caused concern. In response to the fears of dismissal or more subtle means of job loss attributed to outspoken comments, professional organizations and trade unions have set up confidential telephone numbers. This allows staff to raise concerns through a third person, the spokesman of the professional organization or union.

Health care professionals have a responsibility to maintain patient details in a secure place and to respect the privacy of the patient. This may include having to avoid confirming that the individual is receiving treatment from the hospital. Any comment about the effect of care on patients must avoid details that might allow a patient's identity to be revealed.

Ethical issues surrounding the treatment of individuals or groups of patients may be referred to the local ethics committee for confidential advice.

An open atmosphere of discussion, the sharing of problems and a willingness to work on areas of poor quality can only be damaged by a climate of fear and threat of dismissal. Improving the quality of health care and service requires a recognition of the integrity of the individual staff members and trust within the group and throughout the organization. Where staff feel free to 'blow the whistle' they rarely need to do so as the open climate usually enables problems to be solved close to their source.

WORKFORCE PLANNING

It is the job of the manpower planner to balance the demand for staff with its supply – to answer the question 'how many staff should we employ and how should they be deployed?' and then to formulate the appropriate policy; to ensure the supply through appropriate training, recruitment, promotion, retention and return-to-work patterns [1].

In complex systems part of this role falls to the immediate manager who has a greater understanding of the professional's requirements and management strategy.

While most workforce planning systems focus on nurses, an effective system should address all grades and disciplines. It should be influenced by the needs of the patient group, the purpose and philosophy of the hospital.

At ward and hospital level, the methods have developed over the years:

- Matron's assessment – based on intuition and tradition;
- Regional formulae – set by the number of beds and speciality, for funding staff for new buildings;
- Workstudy formulae – based on tasks and fitting patients into defined categories of dependency;
- Nurse time required – calculated on each patient's requirement for nursing care as set out in the care plan.

The use of computer-based care plans allows the fourth method to be performed automatically. If the staff duty rotas are on the same machine, the care hours required can be compared with the staff hours available for each shift. Managers and ward sisters/charge nurses can use the information to deploy staff, to plan staffing levels and resources. It can also be used to identify trends. Some systems are used in conjunction with monitoring the quality of care; however, most of the current systems have had their methodology criticized at one time or another.

Government and independent organizations are reviewing and developing workforce planning systems. The Greenhalgh guide to all the current computer-based nurse-management systems [2] provides a useful starting point. The NHS resource management initiative provided funding to help pay for the pilot nursing systems in acute hospitals.

In developing a workforce strategy for the wards and direc-torate, it is helpful to start by identifying the immediate, medium- and long-term external changes and how they may affect the overall strategy. This includes local demographic projections to see if there will be a workforce available. The drop in the number of school-leavers is well-known. There may be alternative sources such as mature entrants from local industries that are about to close down. New stores or private hospitals may attract staff away from the hospital.

Internal health service changes include the purchaser's plans, which may require new skills from staff. Major capital schemes often need long-term planning.

The changes in professional education programmes, in particular the supernumerary status for student nurses, require replacement with qualified staff and health care assistants. This has implications for recruitment, education and training, as well as morale.

The enrolled (second level) nurse-conversion course will produce more registered nurses after a temporary hiatus while they undertake the course. The manager should consider if there are any who would apply for conversion if help and encouragement were available. The open-learning schemes can also help support more ENs for the same cost as the 1-year course. It is also important to plan the development of those who do not wish to convert so that they feel valued and stay in the team.

The staff budget, number in the post and the skill mix should be examined. Job descriptions and current roles should be reviewed, along with trends and any quality scores. The proportion of staff by grade, gender and part- to full-timers may give clues to work patterns and their relationship to the current quality of care. Retention rates and sickness patterns may indicate the morale of the directorate or a particular ward.

Through looking at staff and workload patterns it may be possible to re-deploy hours to accommodate peaks and troughs in workload, to reduce lengthy overlaps or eliminate outdated procedures to make more effective use of staff time. The recruitment policy should be examined and a retirement/age profile constructed to aid in succession planning.

Staff can be prepared for promotion through education and training such as staff development programmes. Consider local or national 'high-flyer' schemes where money is available to staff with management potential. The directorate might also be able to offer consolidation experience to 'high-flyers' and benefit from their energy and insights.

References

1. Institute of Manpower Studies (1990) *Manpower Planning and Health Care Labour Markets. A Practical Approach,* Session notes, March 1990, Institute of Manpower Studies, University of Sussex, Falmer, Brighton.
2. Greenhalgh & Co. Ltd (1990) *Nurse Management Systems: A Guide to Existing and Potential Products,* Greenhalgh & Co. Ltd, Chatham House, Church Street, West Macclesfield, SK11 6EJ.

Further reading

Ball, J., Hurst, K., Booth, M. and Franklin, R. (1989) *But Who Will Make the Beds?* The Nuffield Institute and Mersey RHA, Leeds University, Leeds.

Carlisle, D. (1989) But who will make the beds? *Nursing Times*, **85**, 37, 18.

Carlisle, D. (1991) Leadership on the fast track to the top. *Nursing Times*, **87**, 1, 25–28.

Clay, T. (1987) *Nurses, Power and Politics*, Heinemann, London.

Gray, A. and Normand, C. (1990) Hidden costs of turnover. *Health Services Journal*, **100** (5225), **November 1**, 1646–47.

Rothwell, C. (1991) Leadership, promoting potential. *Nursing Times*, **87**, 1, 28–30.

X/Y

In the 1950s, McGregor developed two theories to describe the underlying beliefs about the nature of humans that influence managers in the strategies they adopt. He thought managers react to the world through their own perception of it. The two contrasting sets of assumptions were seized upon by his readers as if there was no middle path. This was in contrast to McGregor's own views.

Theory X assumptions about people

These are:

- Humans are inherently lazy and will shun work if they can;
- People must be directed, controlled and motivated by fear of punishment or deprivation to impel them to work as the organization requires;
- The average human prefers to be directed, wishes to avoid responsibility, has relatively little ambition and, above all, wants security.

Theory Y assumptions about people

- For most people the expenditure of physical and mental effort in work is as natural as play and rest;
- Self-control will be exercised in the service of objectives that are accepted by the person;
- Under proper conditions the average human learns not only to accept responsibility but also to seek it;
- The capacity for exercising imagination, ingenuity and creativity exists generally among people.

Since McGregor's time, management theory has developed and the need for flexibility in management styles has been recognized. Organizations have tended to move towards the theory Y view, as it then allows greater use of the talents of the workforce to be made, to innovate and improve the quality of work and its products.

Further reading

McGregor, D. (1960) *The Human Side of Enterprise*, McGraw-Hill, New York.
McGregor, D. (1967) *The Professional Manager*, McGraw-Hill, New York.

Z

ZIZZ

A useful test of good management practice is how well the manager sleeps at night and whether they worry about what is happening in the directorate in their absence.

Some managers forget the night staff. A comparison of the amount of time spent by the manager with the day and night staff could prove interesting. As hospital care continues over 24 hours, regular visits and overlap times need to be planned.

A manager who has responsibility for night staff, such as internal rotation from day to night, should work at least one full night shift a month.

It may help communications if the manager comes on duty early, with a 45-minute overlap with the night staff. This can provide an 'open-door' time when anyone can call, on a 'first come, first served' basis. This way problems or information get discussed soon after they arise.

Many senior sisters (G grade) now have 24-hour accountability for nursing. Experienced sisters may be employed at night to deal with emergencies and to co-ordinate staff development for those on night duty, and sometimes non-clinical services.

Night staff are a valuable asset since back-up services may be poor at night. Examine the speed of response at night. Find out if patients and staff have a long wait for answers to their problems. Do they get told to wait for the day shift to arrive? The same standard should apply no matter what the hour.

Further reading

Duckett, R. (1993) Thirst for knowledge. *Nursing Times*, **89**, 35, 29–31.

Index